THE
ATKINS® 100
EATING
SOLUTION

THE
ATKINS® 100
EATING
SOLUTION

EASY, LOW-CARB LIVING
FOR EVERYDAY WELLNESS

COLETTE HEIMOWITZ

ATRIA PAPERBACK
NEW YORK   LONDON   TORONTO   SYDNEY   NEW DELHI

ATRIA
PAPERBACK

An Imprint of Simon & Schuster, Inc.
1230 Avenue of the Americas
New York, NY 10020

First Atria Paperback edition December 2020

ATRIA PAPERBACK and colophon are trademarks of Simon & Schuster, Inc.

For information about special discounts for bulk purchases, please contact Simon & Schuster Special Sales at 1-866-506-1949 or business@simonandschuster.com.

The Simon & Schuster Speakers Bureau can bring authors to your live event. For more information or to book an event, contact the Simon & Schuster Speakers Bureau at 1-866-248-3049 or visit our website at www.simonspeakers.com.

This publication contains the opinions and ideas of its author. It is intended to provide helpful informative material on the subjects addressed in the publication. It is sold with the understanding that the author and publisher are not engaged in rendering medical, health, or any other kind of drawing inferences from it.

The author and publisher specifically disclaim all responsibility for any liability, loss or risk, personal or otherwise, which is incurred as a consequence, directly or indirectly, of the use and application of any of the contents of this book.

Interior design by Timothy Shaner, NightandDayDesign.biz

Manufactured in the United States of America

1 3 5 7 9 10 8 6 4 2

Library of Congress Cataloging-in-Publication Data
Names: Heimowitz, Colette, author.
Title: The Atkins 100 eating solution : easy, low-carb living for everyday wellness / Colette Heimowitz.
Description: First Atria Paperback edition. | New York : Atria Paperback, 2020. | Includes bibliographical references and index.
Identifiers: LCCN 2020031319 (print) | LCCN 2020031320 (ebook) | ISBN 9781982144241 (paperback) | ISBN 9781982144258 (ebook)
Subjects: LCSH: Reducing diets. | Low-carbohydrate diet—Recipes. | Sugar-free diet—Recipes.
Classification: LCC RM222.2 .H3455 2020 (print) | LCC RM222.2 (ebook) | DDC 641.5/6383—dc23
LC record available at https://lccn.loc.gov/2020031319
LC ebook record available at https://lccn.loc.gov/2020031320

ISBN 978-1-9821-4424-1
ISBN 978-1-9821-4425-8 (ebook)

CONTENTS

PART ONE: How Atkins 100 Works

PART TWO: Putting It All Together: Meal Plans, Low-Carb Hacks, and More

PART THREE: Mouthwatering Low-Carb Recipes for Optimal Energy and Flavor

THE
ATKINS® 100
EATING
SOLUTION

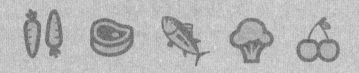

FOREWORD

ROB LOWE

I STARTED LIVING my Atkins low-carb lifestyle when I was in my thirties and realized that I couldn't eat like a teenager anymore. Like many Americans, I knew I had to eat better—my health and my career depended on it. I took a hard look at what I was eating, and I started cutting back on carbohydrates and sugar. Luckily, I love all the foods that make up a low-carb lifestyle: a variety of meats, fish, and chicken; good fats such as those in avocados, nuts, cheese, and olives; lots of colorful vegetables; and even some whole grains. I will admit that bypassing the breadbasket at dinner was tough at first, but now I don't even think about it! I noticed immediately that I had more energy and didn't get that postlunch slump that I used to complain about. After a long day on a film set, I could go for a workout, and I did not need to take a nap. In short, I just *felt* better.

I can guess what you're thinking: "Rob, you've never had a weight problem. Why do you need Atkins?" That, my friends, is the reason this book was written. Atkins 100 is a low-carb, low-sugar approach that pretty much sums up the way I've been eating for years. It isn't just about losing weight; it's about your health and overall wellness. It's about *preventing* weight problems and, even better, avoiding long-term health issues such as type 2 diabetes. It isn't just some short-term fix you "try" for a few months; it's a personalized low-carb approach to eating and an accessible and livable way of looking at food and the integral part it plays in our lives. Atkins 100 is not a diet; it's a lifestyle.

The author, Colette Heimowitz, has been the Atkins nutritionist for more than twenty-five years. She worked with Dr. Atkins in his clinical practice in New York, helping patients with a myriad of health issues—cardiovascular disease and type 2 diabetes, to name two. When it comes to low-carb eating, she knows it all, and she has devoted her life to empowering and educating people about why and how to eat this way. Because let's face it: how we feed ourselves has a powerful effect on our overall health. And if I've learned anything during these last twenty years of living Atkins' low-carb lifestyle, it's that my energy, vitality, and health have been forever changed.

Now, let me be clear: I am not perfect, and I've been known to indulge in a little New York pizza and ice cream. But this is a marathon—not a sprint. This is about progress—not perfection. Everyone can do this, and you *will* benefit from it. If you live this way as consistently as you can, not only will you feel good now, you will feel good later and save yourself from potential future health problems—and have some fun and eat some delicious food while doing it.

In this book, you will learn how to live Atkins 100's sustainable low-carb lifestyle, and, even more important, understand why it's a better way to eat for a lifetime. You will find out how, with the right tips and hacks, plus the more than fifty brand-new low-carb recipes, you can fill your kitchen and your plate with a rich variety of delicious, satisfying foods. Smart shopping, meal planning, and prepping will be laid out for you, and all on a budget. And you'll learn how to make the best choices when you're ordering in, dining out, or eating on the road. You will get a feel for what 100 grams of Net Carbs a day looks like, what it means, and how easy it can be to keep within that range. With Atkins 100, there even is the possibility of a little pizza or a taste of bread, because no food is really off limits. I believe that once you finish reading this book, you will be empowered with the tools you need to thrive and enjoy the Atkins 100 lifestyle.

So here's to you and your health. I'm so glad you're here!

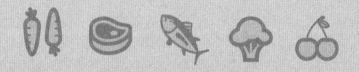

INTRODUCTION

CARBS ARE THE CULPRIT

It's still happening: the standard carb-heavy American diet and out-dated US Dietary Guidelines, which recommend that 45 to 65 percent of your daily calories come from carbohydrates and only 20 to 35 percent from fat, continue to contribute to the twin epidemics of obesity and diabetes.

A 2015 study published in the *American Journal of Clinical Nutrition* analyzed data from 1971 to 2011 to see which macronutrients increased during this epidemic, and it's no surprise: with carb consumption going from just below 40 percent of total caloric intake to 51 percent, carbs are the culprit.

During this period, while fat intake as a percentage of calories consumed declined and protein consumption remained pretty steady, we ate more low-fiber refined carbs, which are inherently devoid of nutrients and love nothing more than to jack up blood sugar levels and store themselves as fat.

Thanks to this, in the United States, 70 percent of adults are now considered obese or overweight; we have the distinction of being the most overweight population in the world, and the *New England Journal of Medicine* recently predicted that half of the US population will be considered obese (not just overweight) in ten years, with one in four severely obese (100 pounds overweight or more). In other not-so-good news, the American Medical Association made it official in 2013 when it classified obesity as a disease. And this new "disease" has the potential to compromise your immune system. New research demonstrates how important building a healthy immunity is and how avoiding unhealthy states such as obesity and type 2 diabetes can help us meet health challenges in the future.

Meanwhile, *52 percent* of the adult population has prediabetes or diabetes, an inability to regulate blood sugar, which is actually carbohydrate intolerance. Even worse, the physical and emotional effects of prediabetes and diabetes go far beyond that. This disease comes at a *huge* cost: if you suffer from it, you can lose your eyesight, and you can lose your limbs. Potentially, it could cost you your life. The American Diabetes Association (ADA) estimated that the cost of treatment of this disease was $327 billion in 2017 and continues to rise.

The good news? Emerging science continues to show the powerful and positive impact nutrition can have on your health, and people are starting to take notice. Whether you're motivated by health issues and the desire to bolster your immune system, you want to reduce your expanding waistline, or you'd just like to feel and look better, our attitudes are changing as we evolve from the low-fat, low-calorie way of eating to consciously controlling the amounts and types of carbs we eat, as shown by the popularity of the keto, low-carb Mediterranean, and paleo diets (to name just a few), all of which are low in carbs and sugar.

THE LOW-CARB CRUSADE

In 1963, a cardiologist named Dr. Robert Atkins immersed himself in the study of the medical benefits of nutrition and learned that controlling carbs instead of calories led to weight loss without significant hunger. He was intrigued, so he and sixty-five of the executives in his private practice went on a low-carb diet; they all lost weight. Buoyed by the success of his own experience with a low-carb diet, in 1972, he published his first book, *Dr. Atkins' Diet Revolution*, which kicked off decades of research and debate within the medical community to determine whether a diet low in carbs and sugar was better for you than a diet low in fat and protein. And you know what? It turned out that Dr. Atkins was right. From Harvard Medical School to the American Heart Association, more than a hundred scientific publications have shown the benefits of living Atkins' low-carb lifestyle, while the media, from the *New York Times* to the *Wall Street Journal*, continue to tout the benefits of low-carb eating as well.

The revolution may have taken a little while to catch on, but the pendulum is swinging in the low-carb direction. It sure seems as though everyone is "doing" keto lately, but this and other popular diet trends, such as low-carb Mediterranean and paleo, tend to be vague in their approaches. Atkins is actually one of the original and more sustainable forms of keto, which gives you a clear-cut way to control your carbs with a wider variety of food than does a hard-core keto diet. I'll show you how later in this book.

It's not surprising that low-carb variations of Atkins keep popping up: you can't go wrong when you choose whole foods that are lower in carbs and sugar. And research continues to support the science behind low-carb eating, with studies showing that beyond weight loss, a low-carb diet can dramatically reduce and even improve a variety of health problems, including prediabetes, diabetes, and cardiovascular disease.

In another encouraging move, the American Diabetes Association has officially recognized a low-carb diet as a viable option for the management of diabetes. But at Atkins, we take this a step further, because we believe that an ounce of prevention is worth a pound of cure. In other words, why wait until you have diabetes when a low-carb diet may help reduce your risk of developing prediabetes and diabetes in the first place?

INTRODUCING THE ATKINS 100 EATING SOLUTION

We know that the path to wellness is not one size fits all, as shown by our current health crisis. Everyone's metabolism processes food in a different way, depending on a person's age, sex, body composition, and overall health, which is why I truly believe in personalized nutrition. When you limit your carbs and consume optimal amounts of protein, nutrient-rich vegetables and fruits, and healthy fats, you control your blood sugar. You experience steady energy levels and less hunger while losing weight or maintaining a healthy weight. How do we know this? It's based on decades of evolving independent, peer-reviewed, published research that has consistently demonstrated improvements in health markers and wellness among people following this type of diet. In addition, decades of working with actual people have shown that Atkins' flexible, easy-to-follow approach that minimizes the consumption of sugar and processed carbs leads to a sustainable low-carb lifestyle. This is why I am excited to introduce Atkins 100 in this book.

While the average American consumes approximately 240 grams of carbohydrates a day, Atkins 100 reduces your carb intake to a doable 100 grams of Net Carbs a day (see page 16 for more on Net Carbs). With Atkins 100, you experience many benefits of a low-carb diet, including increased energy, steady blood sugar levels, and appetite control, as well as improvements to your overall wellness, while enjoying a variety of food.

HOW TO USE THIS BOOK

Just as with Atkins, you can personalize this book to your needs. Start with Part One to learn how Atkins 20, Atkins 40, and Atkins 100 work, skip right to the delicious new low-carb recipes in Part Three, or check out our meal plans and tips for living a low-carb lifestyle in Part Two.

Part One: I will give you an overview of the science behind Atkins, how Atkins works, the basics of carbs, protein, and fat, and how Atkins compares to other popular low-carb and low-sugar diets. Then you'll learn more about Atkins' three low-carb plans, getting all the information you need to determine which approach is best suited for your life: Atkins 20, Atkins 40, Atkins 100.

Part Two: Now that you know how Atkins works and how Atkins 100 can be your everyday eating solution, I'll show you how to curate a low-carb kitchen as well as give you important meal-planning and shopping tips, so when it's time to explore our delicious meal plans, you're ready! You'll find one week's worth of Atkins 100 meal plans, and I'll show you how to modify or, as I like to say, "level down" each meal plan to Atkins 40 or Atkins 20. I will also share my favorite, time-tested low-carb hacks for every occasion, whether you're eating out, at work, on the road, and more.

Part Three: You'll crave these more than fifty brand-new mouthwatering low-carb recipes! Each recipe is designed for Atkins 20, but for the first time ever, I give you easy ingredient options so you can level up the same recipe for Atkins 40 and Atkins 100.

ABOUT ME

I've been with Atkins for more than twenty years, starting when I worked with Dr. Atkins as a nutritionist, and I have helped thousands of patients lose weight and overcome health problems by following a low-carb diet. It has been so fulfilling to be on the cusp of this low-carb trend, which has continued to thrive and change our perception of how we should eat.

Since then, I've been working for Atkins in one capacity or another, observing an advising members of the Atkins community in their weight loss efforts. I travel the country educating people and speaking to the media about a low-carb lifestyle. I've even testified on Capitol Hill during our continual quest to change the US Dietary Guidelines so they are realistic and truly reflect what can actually work for the US population. You may have even read my previous book, *Eat Right, Not Less: Your Guidebook for Living a Low-Carb and Low-Sugar Lifestyle.*

It's fair to say that I'm passionate about anything low carb, not only because I've seen all the science that supports it. I myself have been living a low-carb lifestyle for more than twenty years. There's nothing I love more than hosting family and friends and providing a delicious spread of low-carb food, knowing they will all be asking for the recipes after our meal.

I look forward to showing you how Atkins compares to other popular low-carb diets and why Atkins' low-carb lifestyle is more sustainable. No matter what your goals are, Atkins 100 is your everyday eating solution, an excellent entry point or a way of living once you've lost weight with Atkins 20 or Atkins 40. The ease with which you can move among these plans is what makes Atkins truly personalized nutrition.

If you're ready, so am I! Let's get started.

Colette Heimowitz

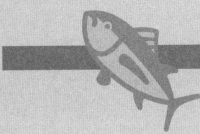

PART ONE

How
Atkins 100
Works

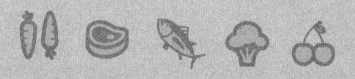

CHAPTER 1

THE FUTURE (AND PAST) IS LOW CARB

AS STEPHEN KING WROTE in *The Colorado Kid*, "Sooner or later, everything old is new again." The same could be said of popular "new" diets such as keto, paleo, and low-carb Mediterranean. These approaches are all derivatives of our lower-carb plan pioneered and made popular by Dr. Robert Atkins in the 1970s.

So let's dig into the science that has fueled today's low-carb renaissance.

Carbs and fat provide fuel for your body, and when carbs are readily available, your body uses them first, converting them into glucose, which is used for energy, and storing any excess as fat. Sure enough, fat storage leads to weight gain, plus the extra carbs cause your blood sugar levels to spike and your energy levels to fluctuate, leading to a nasty cycle of hunger, cravings, and fatigue.

When you limit your carb intake, your body begins to use fat for fuel. After just a few weeks of eating this way, you'll start *burning* fat instead of *storing* it, while feeling full of energy, with less hunger and fewer cravings. The longer you stick with this approach, the more rooted will become the long-term health benefits of a fat-burning metabolism, which will help you avoid spikes in your blood sugar level.

Low-Carb Science Bite

A common misconception about low-carb diets is that if you don't eat enough carbs you will have brain fog and fatigue because your body and brain need glucose (sugar) to function. This is wrong! Other than a few specialized cells (such as red blood cells and some cells in the eye), our bodies are very capable of using fat and ketones for fuel. In fact, your liver is perfectly able to make its own glucose in a process known as gluconeogenesis, providing whatever blood sugar is needed for specialized cells that can't use fat or ketones for energy. Since the inception of Atkins, study after study has shown that not only do people lose weight on low-carb diets, but they sleep better, have more energy, and have no problems with cognition.

LOW-CARB VERSUS KETO: WHAT'S THE DIFFERENCE?

Not to confuse the issue, but a ketogenic diet is a low-carb diet, but not all low-carb diets are ketogenic. Here's why.

- An extreme ketogenic diet (aka keto diet) is quite strict and usually consists of 70 to 80 percent fat, 20 to 25 percent protein, and 5 to 10 percent carbs, which is about 15 to 30 grams of Net Carbs a day.
- Atkins 20 is also considered a ketogenic diet, because you're eating only 20 grams of Net Carbs a day.
- A very-low-carb diet is still considered a ketogenic diet, and you'll eat 50 grams of Net Carbs a day or fewer. Atkins 40 fits the bill here, while providing more variety than a ketogenic diet does.

The bottom line? You can achieve ketosis on both Atkins 20 and Atkins 40. On Atkins 100, you're able to enjoy all the health benefits of a low-carb diet while still eating a full range of delicious food.

What Is Ketosis?

When you burn fat for fuel instead of storing it, as you do on a low-carb diet when you're eating 50 grams or fewer of Net Carbs a day, you have a fat-adapted or keto-adapted metabolism, and you can achieve ketosis (the by-product of fat burning), which is a component of the keto diet.

There's no denying these scientifically based benefits to cutting sugar and limiting carbs, but it can get confusing trying to decipher the difference between all these low-carb approaches. Flip to pages 55–66 to see how Atkins 100 compares and how to modify each of these approaches for your Atkins 100 lifestyle.

Tip: You can find a chart of how Atkins compares to other low-carb diets at www.Atkins.com in the "How It Works" section, under "Compare Diets."

THE PROVEN SCIENCE BEHIND A LOW-CARB DIET

Studies show that a low-carb diet may help you:

- **Lose more weight:** Studies have consistently shown that a low-carb or ketogenic diet can help you lose more weight than a high-carb diet, plus people who follow a low-carb or ketogenic diet had less hunger and found it easier to stick to the diet.

- **Reduce stubborn belly fat:** This kind of stored fat can increase the risk of heart disease, type 2 diabetes, and premature death, but a low-carb or ketogenic diet is a very effective way to lose belly fat.

- **Lower your blood sugar level:** A high-carb diet and poor insulin function can over time lead to a high blood sugar level, which may cause type 2 diabetes, obesity, heart disease, and premature aging. Fortunately, a low-carb or ketogenic diet can help lower blood sugar levels.

- **Drastically reduce insulin resistance:** As with blood sugar, your insulin resistance is directly linked to the quality of your health, risk of disease, and overall metabolic health.

- **Lower triglyceride levels:** Blood triglycerides are an important measure of heart health and show how much fat is in your blood. High levels are linked to heart disease.

- **Increase HDL ("good") cholesterol:** This type of cholesterol plays a key role in helping your body recycle or get rid of cholesterol in the blood, and a high HDL level is linked to a reduced risk of heart disease. One of the best ways to increase your HDL is by increasing your fat intake on a low-carb diet.

- **Lower your perception of hunger:** Typical diets often lead to feelings of constant hunger and deprivation, leading to binge eating or quitting. A low-carb diet has been shown to reduce your hunger more than a low-fat diet does.

- **Boost fat burn during exercise:** A low-carb diet can improve your ability to burn stored body fat instead of glucose during exercise.

- **Reduce epileptic seizures:** A ketogenic diet (high in fat and low in carbs) can help reduce the frequency of seizures in epileptic children, and in some cases it can eliminate seizures altogether. In fact, the ketogenic diet was originally developed in the 1920s specifically to help control seizures in children.

- **Reduce tumor size:** Early-stage research in animals and humans shows that a ketogenic diet may reduce tumor size and help fight cancer.

Metabolic Syndrome's Troubling Trifecta

A diet high in carbs stresses your body, causing spikes in blood sugar, a rush of insulin from the pancreas, and excess fat storage. If this continues over time, your body loses its ability to process carbs and becomes resistant to the insulin rush. The potential result? Metabolic syndrome, a troubling trifecta of health issues characterized by abdominal obesity, decreased ability to metabolize glucose and insulin, and even high blood pressure. It's estimated that nearly one of every three American adults has this condition, which puts them on the fast track to developing type 2 diabetes and triples their risk of developing heart disease. The good news? A low-carb diet has been shown to be extremely helpful in reversing metabolic syndrome. In one study in which people with metabolic syndrome were put on a low-carb diet, the majority of them reversed their condition after only four weeks of dietary changes, even if they didn't lose weight.

MORE ON MACRONUTRIENTS

Though Atkins is low carb, it is most definitely not no carb. From the first printing of *Dr. Atkins' Diet Revolution* in 1972, the intent has always been to *limit*—but not eliminate—carbs. Whole foods, including vegetables, low-glycemic fruits, nuts, and, in later phases, legumes and whole grains, all contain carbs and can be beneficial to your health if your carb tolerance allows it. With Atkins, you'll learn how to identify the carbs that optimize your energy levels and control your hunger, while limiting the carbs that drive your blood sugar level up, which is associated with health risks and weight gain. And you'll learn why it's so beneficial to limit your carbs in general.

Carbs are considered one of three macronutrients, the other two being protein and fat. Each of these macronutrients provides you with calories and is necessary for you to function optimally.

There are two types of carbs that you need to consider: low glycemic and high glycemic. High-glycemic carbs are digested quickly and convert to blood sugar quickly, while low-glycemic carbs are slower to be digested. You should focus on the lowest-glycemic carbs, such as high-fiber colorful vegetables and low-glycemic fruits, such as berries and nuts. Higher-glycemic carbs include grains, cereals, potatoes, breads, and pasta. Higher-glycemic fruits such as bananas and tropical fruits tend to have more naturally occurring sugars. Dairy products also contain carbs, in the form of milk sugars, but higher-fat dairy products contain less milk sugar.

Your metabolism is designed to process 5 grams of glucose at a time, which is equal to about 1 to 2 teaspoons of sugar. If you have more than that circulating in your bloodstream, the excess sugar is first used for energy and what you don't need for energy is stored as fat. Most people probably think this applies to foods such as white rice, white bread, candy, and cookies, but even so-called healthy carbs, such as fruit-sweetened yogurt, your morning smoothie, or a whole wheat bagel, can cause spikes in blood sugar similar to those produced by a candy bar and become stored as fat. We call this the Hidden Sugar Effect. You don't see the excess sugar the food is converting to, but your body does.

Fiber: Your Secret Weapon

Atkins has evolved over the years, based on scientific developments. One important discovery was the role of fiber in carb metabolism. Although fiber is considered to be a carb, it is not digested, unlike carbs that are made up of simple sugars or starches. Fiber actually slows the digestion of other carbs and also slows the rise in blood sugar. That is why we count only the Net Carbs of whole foods (total carbs minus fiber.) For this reason, fiber-rich vegetables are an essential part of Atkins. From the beginning, you'll be eating 12 to 15 grams of Net Carbs of fiber-rich Foundation Vegetables (see page 36) every day.

Why Fiber Is Good for Your Gut

There are two main types of fiber in the diet: insoluble and soluble. Soluble fibers are soluble in water, hence the name. This type of fiber has gelling activity in the large intestine and can help regulate stool frequency. Soluble fiber is found in many foods that you can eat on Atkins, such as nuts and seeds, legumes, and some fruits and vegetables. Insoluble fiber, which is found in many vegetables, adds bulk to the stool and can help if you are suffering from constipation.

The health benefits of fiber are varied, and much of it is likely related to the ability of certain fibers to feed the bacteria that live in the intestines, known as the microbiome. Higher fiber intakes have been linked to a multitude of health benefits, ranging from reduced risk of cardiovascular disease to better digestive health. The fibers that can be broken down by bacteria essentially help stimulate the growth of these bacteria and are referred to as prebiotic fibers. The concept of prebiotics is relatively new, but they have been defined by researchers from the University of Cambridge as "nondigestible food ingredients that beneficially affect the host by selectively stimulating the growth and/or activity of one or a limited number of bacteria in the colon, thus improving host health." When these fibers are broken down by bacteria, they sometimes produce short-chain fatty acids, which provide the cells lining our gastrointestinal tract with energy and also have important roles in the human body such as suppressing appetite, decreasing inflammation, and stimulating immune development. An example of the benefits of fiber to the immune system can be seen in a study in which researchers had study participants swap out high-glycemic, refined carbs for whole grains containing fiber. That swap resulted in an increased production of gut-friendly short-chain fatty acids and a boost to the immune system.

This is why the fiber-rich Foundation Vegetables you eat on Atkins are key to keeping your gut functioning and healthy while limiting their impact on your blood sugar.

How Do You Measure Net Carbs, and What Are They, Anyway?

Net Carbs are the only carbs that matter on Atkins, and they can be calculated by subtracting grams of dietary fiber from total carb grams on a food label. You can download the Atkins Carb Counter for free at Atkins.com. This guide provides the Net Carb counts of practically every food.

Nutrition Facts

1 servings per container
Serving size 1 Shake (325 mL)

Amount per serving

Calories 170

	% Daily Value*
Total Fat 9g	12%
Saturated Fat 2.5g	13%
Trans Fat 0g	
Polyunsaturated Fat 0.5g	
Monounsaturated Fat 6g	
Cholesterol 15mg	5%
Sodium 160mg	7%
Total Carbohydrate 9g	3%
Dietary Fiber 5g	18%
Total Sugars 2g	
Includes 0g Added Sugars	0%
Protein 15g	28%

Vitamin D 0.3mcg	2%
Calcium 240mg	20%
Iron 3mg	15%
Potassium 660mg	15%
Vitamin C 9mg	10%
Niacin 4.5mg	30%
Vitamin B6 0.5mg	30%
Vitamin B12 1.4mcg	60%
Pantothenic Acid 2.5mg	50%

*The % Daily Value (DV) tells you how much a nutrient in a serving of food contributes to a daily diet. 2,000 calories a day is used for general nutrition advice.

Complex Carbs: "It's Complicated"

Though carbs such as whole wheat bread and pasta and grains such as quinoa or bulgur contain fiber and are much better for you than carbs such as white rice and white bread, your body still treats them as, well, carbs—meaning that anything beyond the 2 teaspoons that your body can process at a time will impact your blood sugar. Thank you, Hidden Sugar Effect.

Low-Carb Science Bite

The pancreas is a little organ near the liver and stomach that makes, stores, and releases the hormone insulin in response to increases in blood sugar. Insulin's most recognized function is to restore blood sugar levels to normal by increasing the transport of blood sugar into (mainly) muscle and fat cells. However, insulin actually does much more and is often called the "storage hormone" because it promotes the storage of protein, fat, and carbs. The main example of this is that insulin promotes the storage of any excess carbs we eat as either glycogen (the storage form of carbs in the body) or, if the glycogen tank is full, encourages the conversion of dietary carbs into fat. While insulin promotes nutrient storage, it simultaneously blocks the breakdown of dietary carbs. Think about it this way: when insulin is increased, it puts the brakes on burning fat for fuel and at the same time encourages the storage of incoming food, mostly as fat. Because low-carb diets significantly decrease insulin levels throughout the day, there are significant changes in fat metabolism favoring decreased storage and increased breakdown. Translation: you burn more fat and store less.

CUT THE SUGAR, CURE YOUR CRAVINGS

Sugar addiction is a real thing, causing a vicious cycle of cravings and more cravings, not to mention swings in energy levels and mood, plus weight gain. But going cold turkey may work! Studies published in the journal *Obesity* showed that a low-carb diet may cure your sugar and carb cravings while decreasing your hunger.

Sugar comes in two forms: added sugars, such as sucrose (table sugar), which is added to foods to make them sweeter, and naturally occurring sugars, which are found in fruits, vegetables, grains, legumes, dairy products, and other foods. Though eating a piece of fruit (which also contains fiber and other nutrients) is a smarter choice than drinking fruit juice sweetened with added sugar, any excess sugar that your body can't process will still be converted to fat.

How to Identify Added Sugars

Added sugars go by many names. On a food label, they include:

- *Agave syrup*
- *Brown sugar*
- *Cane syrup*
- *Cassava syrup*
- *Coconut nectar*
- *Corn sweetener*
- *Corn syrup*
- *Corn syrup solids*
- *Dextrose*
- *Fructose*
- *Fruit juice concentrate*
- *Galactose*
- *Glucose*
- *High-fructose corn syrup*
- *Honey*
- *Invert sugar*
- *Lactose*
- *Malt*
- *Maltose*
- *Malt syrup*
- *Maple syrup*
- *Molasses*
- *Raw sugar*
- *Rice syrup*
- *Sucanat*
- *Sucrose*
- *Turbinado sugar*

GETTING TO KNOW THE GLYCEMIC INDEX AND GLYCEMIC LOAD

Glycemic means "relating to sugar," and if you've been paying attention, that's the common theme so far. The higher the glycemic impact of a food, the greater and more rapid effect it has on your blood sugar when you eat it.

Atkins has always been considered a low-glycemic approach, and you've probably heard of the Glycemic Index (GI), which measures the impact of a food on your blood sugar. The GI of a particular food is determined by comparing the effect of a 50-gram portion of that food on your blood sugar to that of a 50-gram standard, such as glucose or white bread. The higher the GI, the faster and greater effect the food's effect on your blood sugar. But the GI does not take into account the portion size you actually eat. A 50-gram portion of carrots is three cups, or six servings, while a 50-gram portion of pasta is only about one-third cup, and in real life, you can see where this goes awry. It's doubtful that you'll be eating three cups of carrots in one sitting, so the GI effect of carrots is probably overestimated, but it's quite likely that you'll be served far more than one-third cup of pasta, so the GI effect of the pasta is under-estimated. This is where the Glycemic Load (GL) of food comes in, as it takes portion size into account and is therefore a much more accurate representation of the effect a food has on your blood sugar levels.

THE POWER OF PROTEIN

Protein contains the amino acids your body needs to repair and regen-erate body tissues and cells. It also preserves lean tissue while promot-ing fat loss, helps keep your hunger in check, and helps maintain stable blood sugar levels. Even better, you burn more calories digesting protein than you burn digesting carbs. You get a lot of bang for your nutrition buck with protein, because you can satisfy your hunger before you're tempted to overeat. On Atkins, you'll eat optimal amounts of protein, typically about 4 to 6 ounces with each meal. You'll find protein in sea-food, poultry, eggs, meat, and dairy products; soy products, nuts, and beans also contain protein, as do as some carb foods.

Meat Has Many Benefits

Although meat has a greater impact on the environment than plant-based foods when it comes to raising it and transporting it, even if you choose to occasionally cut back on it, it's import-ant to point out that it is a nutrient-dense food. When it comes to micronutrients such as copper, zinc, and iron, not only is meat a great source of these minerals, but it's also one of the most bio-available sources—meaning that the forms of these nutrients in meat are easily absorbed by your body. Red meat in particular is known to be a very good source of heme iron, the most bioavail-able type of iron. Another important compound found in meat and other animal products is vitamin B_{12}. In fact, one 3.5-ounce serving of beef contains two-thirds of your daily requirement of vitamin B_{12}, and it's well established that regular consumption of meat lowers the risk of having inadequate B_{12} intake.

One of the more interesting compounds found in the meat (and dairy products, too) of ruminants (this includes cows, sheep, goats, buffalo, deer, and elk) is a type of fatty acid known as con-jugated linoleic acid (CLA). CLA has been demonstrated to have beneficial effects on heart health and insulin sensitivity, and it has also been shown to favorably modulate immune function in humans. In studies in which CLA has been used as a dietary sup-plement, researchers have found that it helps reduce body fat and body weight. Some studies even suggest that CLA helps build lean muscle mass.

WHY YOU NEED TO EAT FAT TO LOSE FAT

Fat is a source of energy and nutrients, is essential for brain function, and helps you absorb fat-soluble vitamins as well as micronutrients in vegetables. As long as you're limiting carbs, the dietary calories from fat are used for fuel and are unlikely to be stored as fat. Though fat contains more calories per gram (9 calories versus 4 calories per gram for carbs and protein), it's hard to overdo it because it takes twice as many calories from low-glycemic carbs as from fat to make you feel full. In addition, fat packs a big punch of flavor, making food appetizing and satisfying.

The right fats, in the right amounts, can turn your body into a fat-burning machine. Here's what you need to know about the different types of fat and where you can find them:

- **Monounsaturated fatty acids (MUFAs):** Found in olive oil and canola oil, as well as in walnuts and most other nuts, as well as avocados. MUFAs are usually liquid at room temperature.
- **Polyunsaturated fatty acids (PUFAs):** Found mostly in oils from vegetables, seeds, and some nuts. Sunflower, safflower, flaxseed, soybean, corn, cottonseed, grape seed, and sesame oils are high in PUFAs, as are the oils in fatty fish such as sardines, herring, and salmon. They are liquid both at room temperature and in the refrigerator.
- **Essential fatty acids (EFAs):** Two families of compounds of dietary fats that your body can't produce on its own. Both omega-3 and omega-6 EFAs are PUFAs essential to your health and well-being. Omega-3s are found in the fat of shellfish and cold-water fish. Omega-6s are found primarily in seeds and grains, as well as in chickens and pigs. Unless you're eating a very-low-fat diet, you are most likely getting more than the recommended amount of omega-6s. Focus on foods or supplements rich in omega-3 fatty acids, such as shellfish, cold-water ocean fish, and fish oil (salmon, tuna, sardines, herring, and anchovies, as well as nonfish sources such as

flaxseeds, almonds, walnuts, and canola oil). Avoid corn, soybean, cottonseed, and peanut oils, which are all high in omega-6s.

- **Saturated fatty acids (SFAs):** Butter, lard, suet, and palm and coconut oils are relatively rich in saturated fats, and tend to remain solid at room temperature. Though the saturated fat in your blood has the potential to gunk up your arteries, dietary saturated fat is fine to consume on a low-carb diet because we know that the body burns primarily fat for fuel, and published research shows that the level of saturated fat in the blood does not increase.

- **Trans fats:** These fats are associated with an increased heart attack risk and have been shown to increase the body's level of inflammation. The good news is that the Food and Drug Administration (FDA) has banned the use of all artificial trans fats in restaurants and grocery stores, noting that this move "could prevent thousands of heart attacks and deaths each year." Though there is a very small percentage of naturally occurring trans fats found in dairy products and beef and lamb, they are not considered harmful.

Get to Know Your Fatty Acids

Though plants contain the omega-3 fatty acid alpha-linoleic acid (ALA), this is not a form of omega-3 that is readily used by your body. The really important omega-3 fatty acids eicosapentaenoic acid (EPA) and docosahexaenoic acid (DHA) are normally obtained only through your diet by eating seafood such as oily fish and shrimp. The anti-inflammatory effects of the omega-3 fats EPA and DHA have been shown in cell culture and animal studies, as well as in studies with humans. These anti-inflammatory benefits are thought to partially explain why these fats have widespread health-promoting effects, especially in reducing the risk of developing heart disease, cancer, and diabetes. Several hundred studies have shown the cardioprotective effects of fish oil, and numerous review studies have supported this. Recent data suggest that EPA and DHA are also crucial for brain function across our life span, and research is under way to see if increasing the intake of these fatty acids can prevent cognitive decline or even depression. Try to eat cold-water fish such as salmon, tuna, cod, sardines, and canned tuna a few times a week. You can also supplement with omega-3 oil, which you can add to smoothies.

Low-Carb Science Bite

The ability to metabolize fat can be measured in research studies, and it should be no surprise that when people go low carb, their ability to burn fat for fuel increases. However, in one interesting study, the researchers asked participants to limit their carbs at breakfast only to an Atkins 100 level, and after four weeks, they found that this alone was enough to dramatically improve the subjects' basal fat-burning ability over the next twenty-four hours. The researchers also observed several other beneficial metabolic effects, such as better blood sugar control. The type of fat might matter, too; if you want more bang for your buck, try adding some monounsaturated fat to your breakfast, such as an avocado, as this seems to boost fat burning the most.

THE *NEW* ATKINS LOW-CARB REVOLUTION IS *YOUR* EVERYDAY EATING SOLUTION

You've seen the powerful benefits you can achieve by eating less sugar and embracing a diet featuring optimal amounts of protein, healthy fats, and fiber-rich carbs. My goal is to help you change the way you eat so that you can enjoy lasting results and make a positive impact on your overall wellness. Coming up, I'll show you how you can jump-start your weight-loss efforts with Atkins 20 or 40 while developing that coveted fat-burning metabolism, and how Atkins 100 is truly the way *everyone* should eat: an easy and delicious way of low-carb eating that you and your family can sustain for life.

With Atkins, low-carb eating is a personalized approach where you can be adventurous while exploring your carb limit, adding in various foods, and discovering what works best for you.

Welcome to Atkins 100. This is your everyday eating solution!

CHAPTER 2

ATKINS 20 AND ATKINS 40: FOR THOSE WHO WANT TO LOSE WEIGHT

Atkins will help you incorporate healthy carbohydrates along with protein and fat into a nutrient-rich, varied, and delectable way of eating for a lifetime.
—*Dr. Robert Atkins*

ARE YOU READY TO LEARN how Atkins' low-carb lifestyle can be customized to fit your needs? Here's a quick overview of Atkins 20, Atkins 40, and Atkins 100 and how Atkins 20 and Atkins 40 can help you achieve your desired weight, setting you up for success so you can follow Atkins 100 for life:

- **Atkins 20** is based on Atkins' original nutritional approach, where you start by eating 20 grams of Net Carbs a day primarily in the form of vegetables, and gradually increase the amount and variety as you reintroduce various foods, starting with low-glycemic carbs and working your way up the Carb Ladder (see page 39). If you are willing to commit to a plan with specific instructions to keep you on track and clear-cut, step-by-step guidelines with little room for guesswork, this is the plan is for you.

- **Atkins 40** sets your carb intake to 40 grams of Net Carbs a day. You still maintain a fat-burning metabolism while having more carbohydrate options and a greater variety of food in controlled portions. This is the way to go if you would like a little less structure than Atkins 20 while still experiencing gradual changes.
- **Atkins 100** is a lifestyle approach that offers flexible eating options and the widest variety of food choices. You eat 100 grams of Net Carbs a day, which makes it easy to feel satisfied while maintaining your weight and healthy lifestyle. Stay tuned, because you'll learn all about Atkins 100 in Chapter 3.

If you're interested in jump-starting your weight loss while enjoying increased energy and stable blood sugar levels and keeping your hunger and cravings under control, try Atkins 20 or Atkins 40.

FIND THE ATKINS PLAN FOR YOU

To start, take this quiz. Even if you think Atkins 100 is the way to go, I highly recommend reading this chapter to learn how Atkins 20 and Atkins 40 work.

Are you curious about what a low-carb lifestyle is all about and would like to make small changes to the way you eat?
Start with Atkins 100.

Do you want to maintain your weight while gradually cutting back on your carbs and sugar?
Start with Atkins 100.

Do you exercise regularly and want to maintain your weight?

Start with Atkins 100.

Do you have fewer than 15 pounds to lose?

Start with Atkins 40 or even Atkins 100, especially if you're young and active.

Do you have 15 to 30 pounds to lose?

Most likely, you'll want to start with Atkins 20, but Atkins 40 is a great option if you'd like to eat a wider variety of food while losing weight at a slower pace.

Do you have more than 30 pounds to lose?

You'll want to start with two weeks of Atkins 20 to get your fat-burning metabolism into gear.

Do you lead a sedentary lifestyle?

Start with Atkins 20 unless you have fewer than 15 pounds to lose, in which case Atkins 40 is fine.

Have you gained and lost and regained weight, i.e., through yo-yo dieting, over the years?

You may have become resistant to weight loss. Either start with Atkins 20 to jump-start your weight loss and discover a new way of eating, or ease into the low-carb approach to eating with Atkins 100 as your starting point, budgeting 25 grams of Net Carbs for each meal and 25 grams of Net Carbs for snacks each day.

Are you over age fifty?

Unfortunately, your metabolism usually slows down over time. Give Atkins 20 or 40 a try for a couple of weeks, and if the pounds start coming off easily, you can gradually level up to a higher carb intake.

Low-Carb Science Bite

Though no one wants their metabolism to slow down, it seems inevitable over time. What's really scary is that excessively strict, low-calorie dieting seems to have the worst effect on metabolism. In a study of participants from the TV show *The Biggest Loser*, researchers found that six years after their dramatic weight loss on the show, "most contestants had regained the weight and body fat that they had lost, but on top of that, their metabolisms had slowed to the extent that they were burning fewer calories every day than they did before their appearance on the show." No wonder they gained the weight back! This is one of the negative side effects of overly strict low-fat, low-calorie diets. Atkins is different—in fact, in a groundbreaking study from Harvard, researchers showed that if participants followed a low-carb approach after losing weight, they had a higher metabolic rate and burned more calories each day than when on a low-fat approach. This is huge, as many people can lose weight, but less than 10 percent are able to keep the pounds off. Once you've gotten away from yo-yo dieting and embrace low-carb living, I am confident it will help you maintain your healthy weight in the long term.

Do you have prediabetes or type 2 diabetes?

Always consult your doctor before starting any new program, especially if you are on medication. Start with Atkins 20 and stay there until you get your blood sugar and insulin levels under control. If you are on blood sugar–lowering medication, you will need to work closely with your doctor to adjust your medication dosage. Your need for blood sugar–lowering medication will decrease dramatically at this level of carb intake, so if you do not have the opportunity to work with a doctor, start with Atkins 100 and work your way down if needed.

Does your waist measure more than forty inches if you're a man or more than thity-five inches if you're a woman, and/or do you have high blood pressure, high triglycerides, and a low HDL level?

You may have metabolic syndrome or prediabetes. Have your doctor check your blood sugar, blood pressure, and insulin levels, then work with your doctor to start Atkins 20 or Atkins 40 and stay with the plan until your blood sugar and insulin levels are under control.

Do you have high triglycerides?

Starting with Atkins 20 or Atkins 40 will help you improve these levels more quickly.

Are you breastfeeding and want to maintain your weight, or are you pregnant?

Start with Atkins 100.

Are you breastfeeding and trying to lose weight?

Atkins 40 gives you a variety of food choices, along with gradual weight loss.

Here's What Atkins 20, Atkins 40, and Atkins 100 Have in Common

- **Net Carbs:** *All you need to do is count the grams of carbs that impact your blood sugar, not total carbs, since the carbs in fiber don't sabotage your body's ability to burn fat.*
- **Protein:** *This mighty macronutrient is essential for fortifying your cells and building muscle, plus it helps keep you full and your blood sugar and insulin at stable levels.*
- **Fat:** *A little goes a long way. Fat adds a huge pop of flavor, while keeping you and your appetite satisfied.*

• **Fiber:** *Fiber has an important role in blood sugar management, and it also fills you up and helps keep your hunger under control.*

Why Low-Carb Food Feeds the Burn

Here's why the fiber-rich, low-carb food you eat on Atkins naturally curbs your hunger and fuels your metabolism:

- *It fills you up.*
- *It keeps your digestion regular.*
- *It takes more energy to digest.*
- *It reduces your cravings.*
- *It is rich in nutrients.*

Why You Need to Keep a Food Journal

No matter what Atkins plan you decide works best for you, a food journal is one of my favorite tools, and research shows that if you use a food journal, you are more likely to achieve your goals than someone who doesn't. In fact, in one study of nearly 1,700 participants, those who kept a record of their daily food intake lost twice as much weight as those who kept no records. A food journal should include the following:

• **What are you eating?** *Write down specific foods as soon as you eat them (don't wait for the end of the day!): what kind of food (or beverages) you are eating or drinking, how was it prepared (baked, broiled, fried, etc.) and any sauces, condiments, dressings, or toppings.*

- **How much are you eating?** *Record your grams of Net Carbs and portion sizes.*
- **When are you eating?** *This can be helpful to determine eating patterns, such as late-night snacking.*
- **Where are you eating?** *At your kitchen table? Standing at your kitchen counter? In front of the computer? In your car? At a restaurant?*
- **What else are you doing while eating?** *Are you working? Watching TV? Talking with a friend or family member?*
- **Whom are you eating with?** *Are you eating with your spouse, your children, a friend, or a colleague, or are you alone?*
- **How are you feeling as you're eating?** *Are you happy, sad, stressed, anxious, lonely, bored, or tired?*

After you've finished a week's worth of food journaling, take a look at what you've recorded. Tracking your daily food and Net Carb intake will give you an honest snapshot of how much and what you are eating, as well as when and why. A food journal can also help you identify trigger foods that have the potential to set off your cravings as well as times of the day when you are most hungry. You can find out how many vegetables you are eating each day, how often, whether you're consuming foods or beverages with added sugars, whether your mood affects your eating habits, and the times of the day when you reach for or crave unhealthy snacks. Using this information, you can set healthy eating goals for yourself.

HOW TO GET STARTED ON ATKINS 20

Atkins 20 is based on the low-carb program first developed by Dr. Atkins and is considered the original keto diet. This approach has helped millions of people achieve their weight loss and wellness goals while giving them a satisfying and delicious way of eating they can stick with for a lifetime, without suffering from crazy cravings or intense hunger.

On Atkins 20, your original, well-constructed low-carb keto diet is split into four levels. On Level 1, you're eating the smallest amount of Net Carbs to burn fat. As you move through Levels 2 and 3, you continue to work toward your goals while gradually balancing and expanding the list of foods you can eat. By Level 4, you're well on your way to experiencing all the benefits of a low-carb lifestyle, eating your maximum amount of Net Carbs while enjoying stable energy levels and maintaining your weight!

HOW LONG DOES EACH LEVEL OF ATKINS 20 LAST?

It depends on your goals! For some, Level 1 may last only two weeks. However, you can safely follow it for much longer if you have a lot of weight to lose or you prefer to lose most of your excess pounds quickly. You can stay at Level 1 until you are 15 pounds from your goal weight if you wish.

Level 2 typically lasts until you're within 10 pounds of your goal weight. However, depending on your goals, you may choose to go to Level 3 sooner. This is also a good option if you are vegetarian or trying to slow down your rate of weight loss.

Level 3 lasts until you've hit your weight loss goal and have kept the weight off for a full month. Waiting a month ensures that you have adjusted to this way of eating and helps you transition smoothly to Level 4.

Level 4 is ongoing and gives you the tools to maintain your goals and live a low-carb lifestyle. This is also the perfect time to move on to Atkins 100.

As you can see, even with Atkins 20, it is truly a personalized approach!

Less Is Not Always More

On Atkins 20, you might lose weight quickly in the beginning, but don't fall into the "less is more" trap I see all the time, where you start cutting even more carbs, thinking that will lead to even faster weight loss. That may cause your progress to stall, and you may even gain weight. Follow Atkins 20 exactly as it is laid out, and you will succeed!

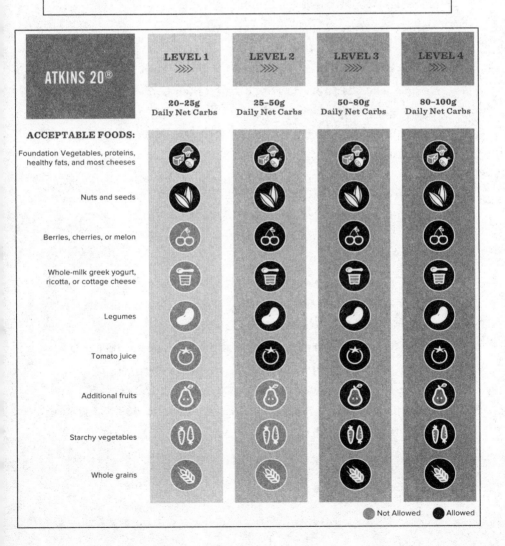

ATKINS 20®	LEVEL 1 ⋙	LEVEL 2 ⋙	LEVEL 3 ⋙	LEVEL 4 ⋙
	20–25g Daily Net Carbs	25–50g Daily Net Carbs	50–80g Daily Net Carbs	80–100g Daily Net Carbs
ACCEPTABLE FOODS:				
Foundation Vegetables, proteins, healthy fats, and most cheeses	●	●	●	●
Nuts and seeds	●	●	●	●
Berries, cherries, or melon	●	●	●	●
Whole-milk greek yogurt, ricotta, or cottage cheese	●	●	●	●
Legumes	●	●	●	●
Tomato juice	●	●	●	●
Additional fruits	●	●	●	●
Starchy vegetables	●	●	●	●
Whole grains	●	●	●	●

● Not Allowed   ● Allowed

Atkins 20, Level 1

Level 1 shifts your body from burning mostly carbs for fuel to burning mostly fat for fuel. You do this by reducing your daily grams of Net Carbs to 20, the minimum amount we recommend to start burning fat and put your body into ketosis.

Think of Level 1 as a way to "cleanse" your system of sugar and high-glycemic carbs. You can follow Level 1 for a minimum of two weeks, but if you like the results and are satisfied with the structure and food choices, you can follow it for longer. It's up to you!

Level 1 Hacks

- **Eat three meals and two snacks a day.** When you eat a filling and delicious meal every three to four hours, you should never feel hungry while following Atkins' low-carb lifestyle. The key is never getting to the point where you're ravenous, as it's much harder to resist your cravings then.

  ....
  Tip: Pair your carb snacks with a fat or protein to minimize the impact on your blood sugar. (Check out our tasty new low-carb snack recipes starting on page 249.)
  ....

- **Eat 20 grams of Net Carbs a day.** 12 to 15 grams of Net Carbs a day come from Foundation Vegetables, and you'll learn how to prepare them in a variety of crave-worthy ways.
- **Eat three 4- to 6-ounce servings of protein a day.** Protein is a natural metabolism and muscle builder, and it come from a variety of sources: meat, poultry, seafood, tofu, eggs, and more.
- **Eat two to four 1-tablespoon servings of fat a day.** Fat is a satisfying and decadent flavor booster to any meal, whether you're cooking with a splash of olive oil or adding a pat of butter to your steamed broccoli.

- **Drink at least eight 8-ounce glasses of water a day.** When you are dehydrated, your body tries to hold on to whatever water is in your body, leading to water retention and bloating. Water helps flush out toxins, aids in digestion, and keeps your skin looking fresh. It's also easy to mistake thirst for hunger. Moral of the story? Stay hydrated!
- **Watch out for added sugars.** These sources of sugar lurk in innocuous places such as pasta sauces and salad dressings, and they will add up over time. Read food labels closely.
- **Use three packets or fewer of sugar substitutes a day.** You've navigated the world of hidden sugars, but what about sugar substitutes? Consume them in moderation, as research shows that they may prevent you from associating sweetness with caloric intake, causing you to crave sweets.
- **Follow the food guides.** It's quite simple. All you need to do is eat foods from the Level 1 Acceptable Foods list on page 283.

· ·

Tip: If you decide to remain at Level 1 for more than two weeks, you can add nuts and seeds.

· ·

Cut the Carbs, Cut the Sugar, Cut the Cravings!

You'd think that reducing your carb and sugar intake would cause your cravings for those foods to go crazy, but the opposite may be true. Research has suggested that a low-carb diet decreases both cravings and hunger.

And for anyone who has been unable to resist a pint of ice cream after a stressful day, this rings true.

Also, women have bigger sweet cravings than men do. Fortunately, another study has shown that after four weeks on a

> *low-carb diet such as Atkins 20 or Atkins 40, cravings for sweets*
> *dropped more for women than men, plus both men and women*
> *lost inches around their waists.*

After two weeks on Level 1, ask yourself:

• Has your energy increased?
• Have your cravings decreased?
• Have you lost weight?

You can stay at Level 1 for longer if you are more than 15 pounds from your goal weight.

If you are happy with your progress and you're ready to add more food choices, it's time to move to Level 2.

What Are Foundation Vegetables?

These vegetables are nutrient dense and fiber rich, and, as the name says, they are the foundation for Atkins' low-carb lifestyle, no matter which level you follow. They keep you full for longer and your energy levels stable and balanced, while packing a powerful nutritional punch. Foundation Vegetables (FV) are primarily salad greens and other raw salad ingredients (see page 94). You can also eat vegetables that are slightly higher-carb (but still permissible) all-stars. Here's where you'll find cancer-fighting cruciferous vegetables, such as kale, Swiss chard, broccoli, and Brussels sprouts; beta-carotene-rich peppers and pumpkin; and lycopene-dense tomatoes, which help protect against prostate cancer.

These two categories of vegetables are an important and tasty part of Atkins from Level 1 on. They're also the first foods you will increase when you gradually add carbs. Eventually you may be able to experiment with starchier vegetables such as potatoes, peas, corn, or beets, but keep in mind that not all vegetables are created equal. These starchier vegetables have a bigger impact on your blood sugar (and waistline), so the key is to get the most bang for your vegetable buck: choose vegetables that provide the most nutrients and fiber with the fewest grams of carbs.

Vegetables: Your Disease-Fighting and Antiaging Secret Weapon

Not only are colorful vegetables an essential part of Atkins, but many studies show that they may:

- Decrease the hardening of arteries
- Help lower cholesterol
- Help prevent inflammation (a factor in obesity, diabetes, heart disease, and Alzheimer's disease)

Atkins 20, Level 2

You're well on your way to embracing a low-carb lifestyle and its sustainable way of eating! You'll start at 25 grams of Net Carbs a day, while gradually increasing your carbs in 5-gram increments. Depending on your Personal Carb Balance (see page 38), you could level off at anywhere between 30 and 100 grams of Net Carbs a day.

Tip: See Appendix B for the complete Acceptable Foods list for Atkins 20, Level 2.

Level 2 Hacks

- **Fill up on veggies.** Keep eating a minimum of 12 to 15 grams of Net Carbs of Foundation Vegetables a day.
- **Add new foods.** Start slow and add new foods from the Acceptable Foods list for Atkins 20, Level 2, one by one, following the Carb Ladder (see Appendix E, "Climbing the Carb Ladder"). If a certain

food triggers a craving, hold off and try another. At this point, depending on how your body reacts, you can start exploring foods such as Greek yogurt, berries, and nuts and seeds to add variety to your meals and snacks.

- **Slow and steady wins the race.** In Level 2, you will slowly increase your carbs in 5-gram increments. This can be done weekly, biweekly, or even monthly. It's up to you! Keep in mind that you're increasing the *variety* of foods you are eating but not the *amount* of food by very much.

- **Tune in to your hunger cues.** Now that you've had time to cleanse your system of the sugar and high-glycemic carbs that were wreaking havoc with your energy and blood sugar level, hopefully you've noticed what causes your hunger or cravings. Your food journal should help you pinpoint the times of the day when you're ravenous, which can help you schedule your snacks and meals to tie into your body's natural hunger cues.

- **Watch out for sweet nothings.** There's nothing like a juicy piece of fruit to satisfy your sweet tooth, but certain fruits may spike your blood sugar or stimulate cravings. They are different for each person, but as you start adding fruits such as berries to your meals and snacks, keep a close eye on how your body reacts to them.

....

Tip: Eat fruit with a little fat or protein to lessen its impact on your blood sugar level (and calm your cravings). Try berries with Greek yogurt or heavy cream or a small piece of melon wrapped in prosciutto.

....

Finding Your Personal Carb Balance

Your Personal Carb Balance is the maximum number of Net Grams of carbs you can consume while continuing to lose weight. This magic number is the secret to steadying your energy level and keeping your appetite and cravings under control while continuing to improve your wellness. Your Personal Carb Balance may well be different from those of other people, as it is affected by your age, gender, activity level, hormonal status, and other factors.

Tip: *The higher the glycemic impact of a food, the greater and more rapid effect it has on your blood sugar when you eat it.*

Climbing the Carb Ladder

The Carb Ladder is a simple tool that helps you add carbohydrate foods as you move past Atkins 20, Level 1, and it also helps prioritize the amount of and frequency with which you might eat those foods. The foods you should be eating most often are on the lower rungs of the Carb Ladder, while you'll eat the foods on the top rungs occasionally or rarely, depending on your tolerance for them. See Appendix E for the foods on each rung of the Carb Ladder and how to introduce new foods and move from one rung to the next.

What Is Carb Creep?

When you start adding back different carbs, sometimes you can lose track of how many grams of Net Carbs you are eating, which means you might regain the pounds you've lost. This is why it's important to increase your carb intake by only 5 grams each week and introduce only one new food at a time. That way you'll immediately notice if a new food is causing cravings. Use your food journal so you can keep an eye on what foods may be the troublemakers.

If you're wondering if you should move to Level 3, ask yourself these questions:

- Are you 10 pounds or fewer from your goal weight? *Move on to Level 3.*
- Are you eating about 20 grams of Net Carbs a day, introducing Level 2 foods, and you're continuing to lose weight without cravings or intense hunger? *Feel free to move on to Level 3 if you're ready to add more variety to your meals. You can always return to Level 2 to jump-start your weight loss again.*
- Do you still have more than 10 pounds to lose, but feel your progress has stalled or you are experiencing cravings and extreme hunger before meals? *Stay at Level 2 until your intense cravings and hunger have subsided.*
- Have you lost weight on Level 1, but your progress has slowed during Level 2, with some foods triggering cravings and hunger? Perhaps you've even gained a few pounds? *You may be very sensitive to carbs, and your Personal Carb Balance may top out at 30 to 35 grams of Net Carbs a day. Be patient and stick with Level 2 for the time being, and ramp up your activity level.*

If you're happy with your results and how you're feeling so far, and you're ready for even more variety in your food choices, it's time to move to Level 3!

Atkins 20, Level 3

You can continue to introduce new carbs in 10-gram increments (or you can stick with 5-gram increments). Carefully watch how your body reacts as you introduce new foods, such as starchy vegetables. The purpose of Level 3 is to help you set the stage for a lifelong way of eating: this is your low-carb lifestyle!

Level 3 Hacks

- **Keep an eye on your cravings.** Continue to add new foods back one by one each day or every few days, depending how you react to that food. At this level, you can start adding starchy vegetables or fruit with more sugar, such as bananas, to your meals and snacks. But if a certain food triggers cravings or uncontrollable hunger, eliminate it for a several days before trying to reintroduce it again.

- **Plateaus require patience.** It's normal for your progress to stall a bit. First make sure that it's a true plateau, meaning you're doing everything correctly (see "Is It a True Plateau?" below). If so, reduce your daily Net Carb intake by 10 grams and wait it out as patiently as you can.

- **Test your tolerance.** What appears to be a plateau may simply be the amount of Net Carbs you can eat to maintain your weight. As with a plateau, reduce your daily Net Carb intake by 10 grams for at least a week. If your weight loss resumes, go up another 5 grams and so forth.

....

Tip: See Appendix C for the complete Acceptable Foods list for Atkins 20, Level 3.

....

Is It a True Plateau?

Weight loss is not always a linear process. It's perfectly natural to experience a few stalls here and there, but if you stick with your plan for a few more days or weeks, you will probably start to see progress. For it to be a true plateau, ask yourself if you meet the following criteria:

- *You've had no weight loss or loss of inches for at least four weeks.*
- *You haven't changed your activity level or made any other significant lifestyle change.*
- *You're not taking any new medications (including hormones) that could interfere with your progress.*
- *You can honestly say you've followed your plan.*

Eight Hacks for Beating a Plateau

First, keep calm and don't give up. Your body isn't like anyone else's, and with time, it will respond if you are patient and consistent. Second, the number on your scale isn't the only way to measure success. Are your clothes fitting better? Do you have more energy? Have your cravings decreased? Are you enjoying satisfying and delicious low-carb meals and snacks? These are all signs that Atkins is working for you! Here are some things you can do to help:

1. *Write everything down that you eat in your food journal. Don't have one? Now is the time to start!*
2. *Reduce your intake of Net Carbs. If you've made it past Atkins 20, Level 1, cut your daily Net Carb intake by 10 grams. You may have stumbled upon your Personal Carb Balance for maintaining your new weight. Once you start seeing progress, start moving up in 5-gram increments again.*
3. *Count all your carbs, including those in lemon juice and sweeteners. Write them down in your food journal.*
4. *Read food labels. Watch out for hidden sugars in sauces, salad dressings, beverages, and processed foods.*
5. *Increase your activity level.*
6. *Make sure you're hydrated. Drink a minimum of eight 8-ounce glasses of water (or other noncaloric drinks such as coffee, tea, or sparkling water) daily.*
7. *Do a reality check on your portion sizes.*
8. *Say bye-bye to booze. If you've been consuming alcohol, back off for a while.*

Ready to move to Level 4? Ask yourself these questions first:

- Are you at your goal weight or adjusted goal weight?
- Have you maintained your weight loss for at least four weeks?
- Are cravings or undue hunger no longer a problem?

If you can answer yes to these questions, it's time to move to Level 4!

Atkins 20, Level 4

Congratulations! By moving through the levels of Atkins 20, you've successfully transitioned from a "low-carb diet" way of thinking to embracing a low-carb lifestyle. You'll be eating the same foods that you've already been eating, but you may be able to experiment with foods that you had unsuccessfully been able to reintroduce earlier and transition to a permanent way of eating.

Level 4 Hacks

- **Go back to basics.** You've made it this far; don't forget the fundamental Atkins tactics:
    - Continue to eat 12 to 15 grams of Net Carbs of Foundation Vegetables every day.
    - Drink eight 8-ounce glasses of water a day.
    - Eat no more than two servings of fruit a day.
    - Consume two to four servings of added fat a day.
    - Eat 4 to 6 ounces of protein at each meal.
- **Get moving.** Take advantage of your increased energy levels and start exercising or take your exercise plan to the next level.
- **Make adjustments as needed.** You may need to tweak your carb intake depending on if you increase or decrease your activity level or overindulge on certain carbs.

• **Watch your portions.** It's fine to "eyeball" portions, but if you notice the pounds creeping on, it's probably time to pay close attention to how much you're eating. It's easy to overdo it on nuts or cheese, so portion them and plan in advance.

> *Tip:* See Appendix C for the complete Acceptable Foods list for Atkins 20, Level 4.

During your Atkins 20 journey, you transitioned from level to level, gradually increasing your carb intake until you might be eating 80 to 100 grams of Net Carbs a day. By gradually reintroducing foods one by one, you have learned which foods, if any, might derail your progress, and you know which foods you can live without and which ones you love but must eat in moderation. You have learned to listen to your hunger cues and how to respond to cravings, and you've seen the powerful impact that reducing your carb intake to 20 Net Grams a day has on your energy levels and your health.

Level Up or Level Down: It's Your Choice

As you've learned so far with the different levels of Atkins 20, moving to the next level is personalized to the progress you are making. If you feel your weight loss is stalled, you can always level down. You can also level up between Atkins 20, 40, and 100, and we've made it even simpler with our Atkins meal plans on pages 100–107, which are customized for each level.

HOW TO GET STARTED ON ATKINS 40

On Atkins 40, you reduce your Net Carb intake to 40 grams a day. You are still burning fat for fuel, and you can achieve ketosis on this more flexible form of a low-carb keto diet, but you are able to eat a variety of foods of your choice, right from the beginning.

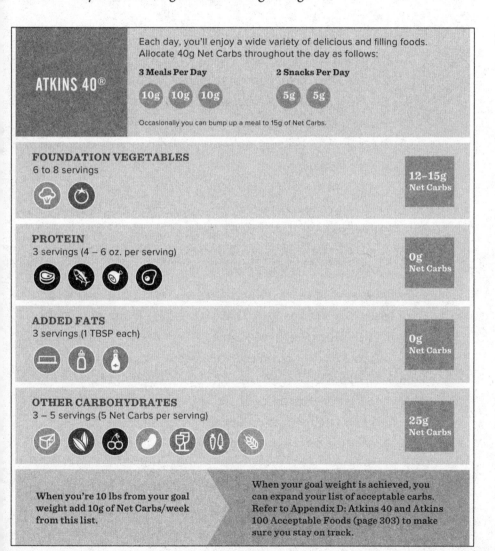

Atkins 40 Hacks

- Unlike in Atkins 20, you don't move through levels as you intro-
duce new foods on Atkins 40 because you can eat a variety of foods
right from the beginning, but just as on Atkins 20, you:
  - Eat 12 to 15 grams of Net Carbs of Foundation Vegetables
every day.
  - Drink eight 8-ounce glasses of water a day.
  - Eat no more than two servings of fruit a day.
  - Consume two to four servings of added fat a day.
  - Eat 4 to 6 ounces of protein at each meal.
- **Know your limits.** Though you can eat a variety of foods on Atkins
40, some foods inherently do you no favors in achieving your
goals. Try to limit or avoid:
  - Foods containing 5 grams or more of added sugars
  - High-glycemic carbs such as white rice and anything contain-
ing white flour
  - Foods that might trigger cravings
  - Foods containing hidden sugars, especially processed foods
- **Prioritize your portions.** If you look at the Acceptable Foods lists
on pages 283–309, you'll see that some food portions are smaller
than others. These foods are higher in carbs and lower in fiber. By
eating smaller portions, you can make the most of your 40 grams
of Net Carbs a day.
- **Give yourself a jump start.** If you're pleased with Atkins 40 but
would like to see speedier results, try these hacks:
  - Reduce the daily amount of Net Carbs you are eating by 5 or
10 grams.
  - Increase the amount of fat you eat and decrease the amount of
protein you are eating if you're eating more than 4 to 6 ounces
of protein per serving.
  - Increase your activity level.

– Look at the higher-carb foods you've eaten lately and swap them for foods higher in fiber and lower in carbs or cut back on your portions of higher-carb foods.

....

Tip: *See Appendix D for the complete Acceptable Foods list for Atkins 40.*

....

Tip: *Ready to get started? See pages 100–107 for one week of meal plans customized to Atkins 40.*

....

What About Happy Hour?

I don't recommend drinking while on Atkins 20, Level 1. On Atkins 40, try to wait two weeks until your body gets into its fat-burning zone. After this, if you wish, you can drink alcohol in moderation. Keep in mind that your body will burn alcohol before fat, so it could slow down your progress. Stick with low-carb beer or a glass or two of wine or spirits such as scotch, vodka, or gin. Watch the sugar in your mixers. Seltzer, diet tonic water, and diet soda are fine, but juices, tonic, and nondiet soda do contain sugar. Just remember, all the carbs in your drinks count, too.

MOVING ON TO ATKINS 100

Now that I've shown you how Atkins 20 and Atkins 40 work and how you can customize these plans to achieve your goals, it's time to learn about Atkins 100, your secret to low-carb living for everyday wellness.

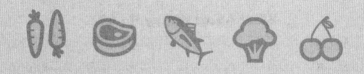

CHAPTER 3

ATKINS 100:
YOUR EVERYDAY
EATING SOLUTION

I really regret eating healthy today.
—*Said no one ever*

I'VE SHOWN YOU THE HARD FACTS about how the US Dietary Guidelines have totally let us down. Reducing your carb intake has the power to increase your energy and control your hunger while having a huge impact on your overall wellness. And this is exactly where Atkins 100's personalized and sustainable approach comes in and why *everyone* should be eating this way: women and men, your family and friends. With Atkins 100 you get to eat a wide variety of foods from all food groups.

Are you ready? Here's how Atkins 100 works:

- Eat 100 grams of Net Carbs a day.
- As with Atkins 20 and Atkins 40, try to eat a minimum of 12 to 15 grams of Net Carbs a day of Foundation Vegetables.
- As for the remaining 85 grams of Net Carbs, don't eat them all at one meal, but distribute them evenly throughout the day. To start, you can take your pick from the Acceptable Foods list in Appendix D.

- Eat three 4- to 6-ounce servings of protein a day.
- Eat two servings of added fat a day, such as a pat of butter or a tablespoon of olive oil or salad dressing.
- Here are some easy ways to spread out your daily 100 grams of Net Carbs:
  - Have three meals a day of 25 grams of Net Carbs (see pages 181, 203, and 225 for Atkins 100 breakfast, lunch, and dinner recipes).
  - Have two snacks a day of 10 to 15 grams of Net Carbs (see page 249 for Atkins 100 snack recipes).
  - Make high-fiber food choices to help you avoid the spikes in blood sugar that tend to affect your blood sugar level over time.

What are the differences among Atkins 20, Atkins 40, and Atkins 100? On Atkins 100, you reduce your fat intake from 60 percent to 70 percent of your total calories to about 50 percent of your total calories while increasing your carb intake. Your protein intake remains the same!

. . . .

Tip: The Acceptable Foods list provides you with a general direction of what to eat, but you may find other carbs not on the list that are also perfectly acceptable, as no food is really off limits on Atkins 100, although I suggest minimizing your high-sugar food choices. Your best bet? Choose carbs that are high in fiber, which will naturally satisfy your appetite before you start overeating.

. . . .

Tip: Do you remember how to calculate Net Carbs? It's simple! Just subtract the grams of fiber from Total Carbohydrates on a food label. As far as packaged foods go, just subtract fiber, as well as sugar alcohol (including glycerin), from Total Carbohydrates to calculate Net Carbs.

. . . .

What Are Sugar Alcohols?

Sugar alcohols come in the form of ingredients such as allulose, glycerin, mannitol, sorbitol, xylitol, erythritol, isomalt, lactitol, and maltitol. Sugar alcohols provide a sweetness and mouth-feel similar to that of sugar, without the calories and unwanted metabolic effects. Sugar alcohols are not fully absorbed by the gut, which means that they provide roughly half the calories that sugar does. Thanks to this incomplete and slower absorption, they have a minimal impact on blood sugar and insulin response. Because of this, sugar alcohols don't significantly interfere with fat burning.

Tip: A snack keeps your metabolism buzzing along, burning calories for energy, instead of going into starvation mode, when it slows down and hoards energy and cravings hit. Whether you call it a minimeal or a snack is up to you, but go for it.

Tip: Eat protein and/or fat with carbohydrates to slow down the rate at which your blood sugar rises.

Quality Versus Quantity

Did you know that the average American consumes 240 grams or more of carbohydrates a day, very often in the form of the high-glycemic variety? With Atkins 100, you are changing the quality of the carbs you are eating, with a focus on fiber-rich, low-glycemic carbs.

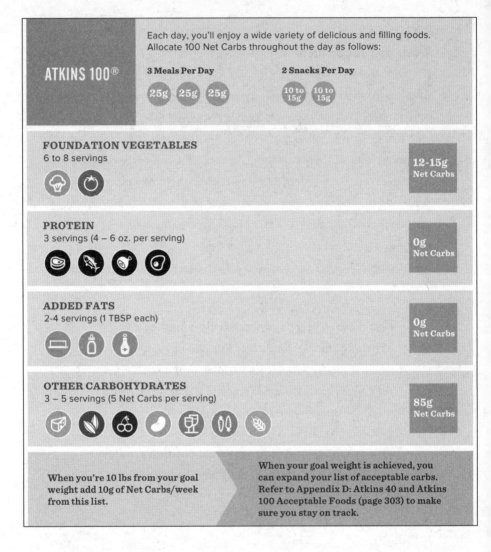

Atkins 100 Hacks

These time-tested hacks are your secrets to success on Atkins 100!

- **Count your Net Carbs.** This will help keep you in check. Keep reading, because this goes hand in hand with portion control.
- **Eat primarily whole foods.** Shop the perimeter of the grocery store for staples; here you'll find fresh vegetables, nuts, and fruits in the

produce section; meat, poultry, and fish at the butcher counter; plus cheese, Greek yogurt, and eggs in the dairy section. (Learn more about my favorite shopping tips on pages 83–84.)

- **Stay away from sugar, white flour, and other junk foods.** Avoid the snack and candy aisles!
- **Don't go more than four to six waking hours without a meal or snack.** This will keep your metabolism humming, your blood sugar level stable, and your hunger in check.
- **Practice portion control.** See the Acceptable Foods list in Appendix D for portion sizes and "How to Eyeball Portion Sizes" on page 76.
- **Choose quality over quantity.** You could easily blow a 25-gram Net Carb "meal" on a bag of chips when you can be savoring a serving of satisfying and delicious Moroccan Chicken Mason Jar Salad (page 209).
- **Exercise regularly.** Combining exercise with Atkins 100 is a win-win approach. See more on the benefits of exercise and workout suggestions on page 67.
- **Drink a minimum of eight 8-ounce glasses of water a day.** Water does wonders for your digestion, your skin, and hunger control.
- **Never let yourself gain more than five pounds.** If you're gaining weight on Atkins 100, it might be time to take a closer look at what you're eating. See page 66 for my tips.

Booze on Atkins 100

You may drink in moderation as long as you remember that you need to count alcohol carbs, too. Consider drinking spirits neat or on the rocks with a citrus twist, a light beer, or a glass of wine with dinner. Beware of mixers such as juice or soda that could contain hidden carbs.

No More Yo-yo Diets

If you have a history of yo-yo dieting, you likely know what it feels like to struggle with a restrictive program, quit out of frustration, and return to your old way of eating. If this is you, stick with Atkins 100's flexibility and wider food choices. From here you can test the waters of this new way of eating and reducing your carbs, and then you can see how low you can comfortably go without losing your focus and commitment.

Follow the Rule of 5

If a food has 5 grams or more of fiber, it's a good choice. If a food has 5 grams or more of total sugars or 5 grams or more of added sugars, put it back on the shelf.

GETTING BACK TO THE GLYCEMIC IMPACT

The glycemic impact of a food is a theme you'll keep reading about throughout this book. The higher the glycemic impact of a food, the greater and more rapid effect it has on your blood sugar when you eat it. Choosing foods with a lower glycemic impact is the secret to maximizing your success and satisfaction with Atkins 100. For example, whole vegetables and most fruits have a smaller glycemic impact than fruit juices do.

Another trick to lowering the glycemic impact and slowing down the onset of hunger is to combine dietary fiber with dietary fat and protein. Eating half an apple by itself may raise your blood sugar, but a slice of cheddar cheese or some peanut butter eaten with it will slow the entry of the apple's naturally occurring sugar into your bloodstream. The same goes if you pair a serving of berries with a dollop of heavy cream or Greek yogurt.

Your goal is to look for the least processed and most fiber-rich food choices you can make. The Acceptable Foods list in Appendix D can help guide you. If you look at the Acceptable Foods list, you'll see that 2 tablespoons of chickpeas have 5 grams of Net Carbs, while you can eat 10 tablespoons of edamame, which also weigh in at only 5 grams of Net Carbs, meaning that the chickpeas have a greater impact on your blood sugar than edamame does. The Carb Ladder in Appendix E can also be your guide, as it starts with foods with the lowest glycemic impact— Foundation Vegetables—on rung 1 and continues to whole grains on Rung 10. What's most important is to make smart and good-quality carb choices that will give you the most bang for your glycemic buck.

ATKINS 100, YOUR WAY: CUSTOMIZING ATKINS 100 FOR OTHER EATING APPROACHES

The wonderful thing about Atkins 100 is that this way of eating complements a variety of other popular diets. Whether you're passionate about paleo, devoted to the DASH diet, or very vegetarian, each of these approaches can go hand in hand with Atkins 100. No matter what diet you choose, counting carbs can be your gold standard and integrated into your consideration for long-term success and overall wellness. Here's how Atkins 100 can be the blueprint that you can adjust to meet the standards of lower-carb versions of six popular diets.

To start, eating at least 12 to 15 grams of Net Carbs of Foundation Vegetables a day complements each of these diets perfectly. And like Atkins 100, these diets focus on cutting back on sugar and processed foods.

DASH Diet

DASH, which stands for Dietary Approaches to Stop Hypertension, is a low-sodium, low-fat, high-fiber approach that was developed to help lower blood pressure and cholesterol. One major tactic of the DASH diet is to consume fruits and vegetables that contain nutrients that help lower blood pressure, such as magnesium, potassium, and other phytochemicals. The meats consumed are primarily lean poultry, fish, and seafood. The diet limits sodium, red meats, sweets, sugary beverages, and anything containing elevated sodium levels, such as frozen meals, salty snacks, and fast food.

Your Atkins 100–Style DASH Diet

Though the DASH diet does not have a set macronutrient range, if you were to follow it, about 55 percent of your daily calories would come from carbs, which is quite a bit more than what you eat on Atkins 100. Therefore, the easiest way to adapt the DASH diet to Atkins 100 is to eat smaller portions of whole grains, while the majority of your carbs come from fruits and vegetables. Focus on eating lean meat and fish and more plant-based proteins and using fresh herbs and spices instead of salt. Dairy products higher in fat tend to contain less sugar and are more satisfying because of their fat content, and they can be eaten on an Atkins 100 version of the DASH diet. In fact, a study published in the *American Journal of Clinical Nutrition* tested the effects of the traditional DASH diet and a modified DASH diet using high-fat dairy products, and the authors of this study concluded, "the results of this study indicate that modification of the DASH diet to allow for more liberal total and saturated fat intake in conjunction with moderate limitation of carbohydrate intake, primarily from fruit juices and sugars, results in lower concentrations of triglycerides and VLDL particles, with no increases in total or LDL cholesterol and no attenuation of the favorable blood pressure response to the standard DASH diet."

Atkins 100–Style DASH Diet Hacks

- Manage your portions of whole grains by replacing half a portion of brown rice with cauliflower rice or half a portion of whole grain pasta with zucchini "noodles."

- Choose lean cuts of beef such as sirloin or tenderloin.
- Go for lean sources of poultry such as skinless chicken or turkey breasts, as well as lean white fish, such as cod, haddock, pollock, flounder, halibut, tilapia, and orange roughy.
- Pick plant-based proteins such as tofu and plant-based crumbles and burgers (read more about plant-based "meat" on page 174).
- Boost your protein with low-carb nuts and seeds such as pepitas and hemp nut seeds, which are also healthy sources of omega-3 fats.
- Select vegetables that are higher in protein, such as avocado, bok choy, broccoli, salad greens, and spinach.

Meal Tip: For an Atkins 100–style DASH diet breakfast, try Spinach, Asparagus, and Charred Scallion Frittata (eliminate the salt) on page 211.

Intermittent Fasting

Intermittent fasting (IF) means cycling between periods of fasting and eating, with fasts ranging from sixteen hours to twenty-four hours or more. The idea behind IF is that it lowers your insulin levels so that your body releases stored fat and burns it for fuel. Hypothetically, no food is forbidden on IF, but most IF fans tend to do it in conjunction with a low-carb or keto diet.

Atkins 100 and Intermittent Fasting

Atkins 100 helps you naturally control your blood sugar level and appetite, but if you'd like to try a twelve- or sixteen-hour fast or longer, stop eating at 7 p.m. and then give your body a reset and your digestion a break. Whether you decide to break your fast with a meal at 7 a.m. or you stretch it until 11 a.m. or noon, simply follow Atkins 100's guidelines of three meals of 25 grams of Net Carbs each plus a couple snacks with 10 to 15 grams of Net Carbs each during your eating window.

Atkins 100–Style Intermittent Fasting Hacks

- Stay hydrated. Be sure to drink lots of water and calorie-free drinks such as herbal tea. A soothing herbal tea, such as chamomile, is actually a great "nightcap" before bed.
- Some people have a fat-only meal within the fasting window, usually in the form of coffee blended with coconut oil or medium-chain triglycerides (MCTs) oil and grass-fed butter, with the thought that the combination of caffeine and these specific fats naturally boosts energy and alertness while curbing cravings.
- Gently reawaken your digestion from longer fasting periods with a drink such as a smoothie or a cup of savory bone broth.
- Atkins 100's nutrient-dense eating approach featuring optimal protein, high-fiber veggies, low-glycemic fruits, nuts, and seeds, and healthy fats will naturally balance your blood sugar levels after your fasting period.

Energy-Boosting Fat Facts

Medium-chain triglycerides (MCTs) break down in the body and are used primarily for energy production, instead of being stored as body fat. Coconut oil contains MCTs. Lauric acid makes up the majority of the MCTs in coconut oil and has been shown to have a favorable impact on serum cholesterol levels.

Meal Tip: For an Atkins 100–style IF snack, try the "Mexican Hot Chocolate" Smoothie on page 194.

Curious About Keto? Atkins May Be
the Better Keto Diet

Ketogenic diets were first used by physicians in the 1920s as a treatment for epilepsy. Dr. Atkins introduced the concept of ketosis to the general public in 1972 in his first book, Dr. Atkins' Diet Revolution. *In simple terms, if you restrict your carbohydrate intake, your body will start to burn fat as fuel. When your body goes into ketosis, your liver produces ketones, which provide an alternate fuel source for the brain, have anti-inflammatory activities, and act as a mild appetite suppressant.*

Similar to a low-carb diet, the keto diet activates your body's fat-burning metabolism by restricting carbs. On a standard keto diet, 75 to 90 percent of your daily calories come from fat, 5 to 20 percent come from protein, and less than 5 percent come from carbs, for a total of about 15 to 30 grams of Net Carbs a day. Unless you are trying to control seizures, the high level of fat consumption on the keto diet may not be necessary and may be difficult to sustain. This is why keto can be confusing, because there are so many definitions and philosophies.

Meanwhile, you can still achieve and maintain the fat-burning state of ketosis by consuming 40 grams of Net Carbs or fewer a day, with about 65 percent of your daily calories coming from fat, as you do on Atkins 20 or Atkins 40, as follows:

- *Atkins 20: Fat: 60 to 70 percent, protein: 20 to 30 percent, Net Carbs: 5 to 10 percent*
- *Atkins 40: Fat: 55 to 65 percent, protein: 20 to 30 percent, Net Carbs: 10 to 15 percent*

A well-constructed keto diet with adequate fiber from vegetables, healthy fats from avocados, olive oil, and butter, and moderate (not excessive) protein intake has been studied in peer review clinical trials for the last four decades and shown to be safe and effective. Sound familiar? But with Atkins, you have structured, clear-cut levels to find your Personal Carb Balance for weight loss and maintenance, plus all of the benefits of a keto diet without the rigid restrictions of high fat and very low carb intake. Eventually you have more flexibility, since you can add some nuts and low-glycemic fruits such as berries and melon, as well as root vegetables.

Although Atkins 100 is out of ketosis range for most people, if you would like to follow a well-constructed, sustainable keto diet, try Atkins 20 or Atkins 40. Emerging science continues to show that this low-carb, low-sugar, keto approach continues to be a healthy, balanced way of eating and living, and Atkins may just be the better keto diet!

Mediterranean Diet

This diet is based on what people tend to eat in Greece, Spain, Italy, and France. You eat vegetables, fruits, nuts, seeds, legumes, potatoes, whole grains, breads, herbs, spices, fish, seafood, and extra-virgin olive oil. You also eat poultry, eggs, cheese, and yogurt in moderation, and you rarely eat red meat. You avoid sugary beverages, added sugars, processed meat, refined grains, refined oils, and other highly processed foods.

Your Atkins 100–Style Mediterranean Diet

The biggest deviation from the normal Atkins 100 approach will be limiting foods such as butter, dairy products, and red meat and also cutting back on processed meats. The typical Mediterranean diet contains more carbs than Atkins 100 does, but the carbs are typically from low-glycemic, fiber-rich sources, so the biggest adjustment is consuming smaller portions of Mediterranean diet–friendly carbs and keeping your Net Carbs at 100 per day. Your remaining 85 grams of Net Carbs can easily consist of legumes and whole grains (think beans, lentils, and fiber-rich whole grains such as farro), as well as poultry, salmon a few times a week, and even some delicious snacks such as veggies and hummus or a handful of almonds with olives.

Atkins 100–Style Mediterranean Diet Hacks

- Swap mashed potatoes for mashed cauliflower or do a combination of both. You can also do a cauliflower mash with mashed white beans, such as cannellini.
- Swap brown rice for cauliflower rice (or a combo of both). (See the recipe for Cauliflower Rice with Butter and Chives on page 183.)
- Swap pasta for zucchini noodles or a combo of both.
- Watch your serving sizes of beans (½ cup of black beans has 13 grams of Net Carbs). See Appendix D for a full list of legumes and whole grains and their serving sizes and grams of Net Carbs.

Meal Tip: For an Atkins 100–style Mediterranean diet dinner, try Roasted Salmon with Crushed Green Olive, Lemon, and Fennel Salad on page 226.

Paleo Diet

This is based on eating whole foods from food groups our hunter-gatherer ancestors would have eaten during the Paleolithic Era. They include grass-fed beef, pasture-raised poultry and eggs, wild-caught fish and seafood, fresh fruits and vegetables, seeds, nuts, and unprocessed oils. The strictest interpretation of the paleo diet eliminates all dairy products, cereal grains, legumes, refined sugars, and processed foods.

Your Atkins 100–Style Paleo Diet

On a typical paleo diet, about 35 percent of your daily calories come from carbs, which tends to be a little higher than we recommend with Atkins 100. So the first step in making Atkins 100 paleo friendly is to make sure you don't overeat paleo-friendly carbs (such as sweet potatoes, fruits, and cassava). After getting your Foundation Vegetables for the day, base your remaining 85 grams of Net Carbs around meals featuring grass-fed beef, poultry, fish, and seafood, plus snacks of fresh vegetables and fruits, nuts, and seeds.

Atkins 100–Style Paleo Diet Hacks

• Watch the grams of Net Carbs in paleo-friendly carbs such as sweet potatoes. For example, half a sweet potato contains 10 grams of Net Carbs. See Appendix D for a full list of starchy vegetables and fruits and their serving sizes and grams of Net Carbs.

• Turnips are a lower-carb alternative to sweet potatoes and potatoes, and they are a staple on the paleo diet. You can make turnip "fries" or roasted turnips.

• The paleo diet does not include legumes, grains, pasta, or bread, so you can do low-carb swaps of cauliflower rice for rice and zucchini noodles for pasta.

• Season your food with sea salt, garlic, and spices such as turmeric, rosemary, thyme, and chili powder, as well as fresh herbs.

> **Meal Tip:** For an Atkins 100–style paleo lunch, try Prosciutto Chicken with Lots of Greens on page 229.

Vegetarian Diet

On a vegetarian diet, you eat vegetables, grains, legumes, nuts, seeds, and fruit, and you eliminate meat, poultry, fish, and seafood. Vegans take it a step further by not eating *any* foods that come from animals, including dairy products and eggs.

Atkins 100 for Vegetarians and Vegans

The key is to make sure you get adequate protein intake as well as B vitamins, including vitamin B_{12}, which is essential for your brain and nervous system to function and is found only in animal foods, such as cow's milk and eggs (in addition to meat). As far as protein is concerned, try vegetarian proteins such as tofu or tempeh, as well as eggs, Greek yogurt, and cheese if you're not vegan. For vegans, your protein will come from plant protein in the form of nuts, beans, soy "burgers," tofu, and plant-based products such as veggie "bacon," "sausage," and "burgers," and you may need to add fortified nutritional yeast flakes, fortified soy milk, and fortified cereals to boost your B_{12} intake. Get your fill of healthy fats from avocados, nuts, soy products, and vegetable oils such as olive oil. Make your snacks filling and satisfying with a combo of high-fiber veggies and nuts and seeds. Although they are vegetarian and vegan, you should try to avoid high-glycemic carbs such as white bread, rice, potatoes, and baked goods and count your daily carbs to remain in the 100 Net Carbs range.

Atkins 100–Style Vegetarian and Vegan Diet Hacks

- You can add or swap hemp hearts and pepitas for grain-based options such as steel-cut oatmeal to decrease your carbs and increase your protein. A quarter cup of steel-cut oats has 12 grams of Net Carbs. Try 2 tablespoons steel-cut oats (6 grams of Net Carbs) plus 2 tablespoons hemp hearts (0 grams of Net Carbs) or 2 tablespoons hemp hearts (0 grams of Net Carbs) and 2 tablespoons chia seeds (1 gram of Net Carbs).
- Turn to page 177 for more suggestions for plant-based dishes and pages 172–174 for tips on boosting the veggie content of any dish.

> **Meal Tip:** For an Atkins 100–style vegetarian dinner, check
> out the Vegetarian Ramen Zoodle Bowls on page 227.

Whole30

This thirty-day diet focuses on whole foods and the elimination of sugar, alcohol, grains, legumes, soy, and dairy products. It is similar to but more restrictive than the paleo diet, as you can't eat natural sweeteners such as honey or maple syrup or some of the low-carb baked goods you can eat on the paleo diet. You can consume vegetables, fruits, unprocessed meats, poultry, seafood, eggs, nuts and seeds, oils, and coffee. The idea is that you learn how your body responds to certain foods by eliminating them and then slowly reinstating them.

Your Atkins 100–Style Whole30

Consider Whole30 as a more restrictive version of Atkins 100 but still with a low-carb and low-sugar focus. Since your 85 grams of Net Carbs won't be coming from grains or legumes, you'll need to get creative with plenty of fruits, veggies, nuts, and seeds, in addition to protein in the form of meat, seafood, and poultry. Alcohol also isn't allowed on Whole30, so you can think of this as a good time to do a thirty-day alcohol detox. See how your body reacts if you decide to add back some grains, legumes, soy, and dairy products or the occasional adult beverage after thirty days.

Atkins 100–Style Whole30 Hacks

- Whole30 may be a good way to counteract a raging sweet tooth or as a reset after the holidays, a vacation, or an extended pandemic quarantine.

- Berries are a low-glycemic, low-sugar Whole30 choice that you can eat for dessert or pair with nuts for a snack.
- Aim for a serving of vegetables with every meal. Balance out starchier, nutrient-dense veggies such as winter squash, sweet potatoes, and beets with Foundation Vegetables such as leafy greens, asparagus, artichokes, and mushrooms.

A Low-Carb Detox?

Detoxification is actually a normal physiological process that occurs every day in your gut, liver, and kidneys. These organs are extremely important for helping remove excess environmental contaminants from your body. Though some cleanses or detox programs suggest drinking celery juice 24/7, this doesn't really make sense. If you are looking to do a cleanse or detox, what you'll want to do is eat in a way that boosts the health of your organs that handle detoxification, and this is where the Atkins 100 approach works perfectly! Cut out sugars and refined carbs to support the health of your liver; increase your fiber intake if you want to help give your digestive system a detoxifying boost. Plus, some research has shown that if you increase your intake of essential minerals, they seem to compete with heavy metals in your gut for absorption and ultimately reduce your exposure to these harmful compounds. So opt for consuming foods that are good sources of essential minerals, such as dairy products for calcium and nuts for copper and zinc.

Meal Tip: For an Atkins 100–style Whole30 meal,
try Coconut Curry Squash Soup on page 208.

Gaining Weight on Atkins 100? Here's What to Do

Though Atkins 100's focus is on improving your overall wellness, not weight loss, if you do start putting on a few pounds while doing Atkins 100, you might want to make these adjustments:

- *If you aren't doing so already, start counting your daily grams of Net Carbs.*
- *Take a hard look at the quality of your meals and snacks. Are you going overboard on naturally occurring and added sugars?*
- *How are your portions? Review the Acceptable Foods list in Appendix D on page 303 and "How to Eyeball Portions Sizes" on page 76.*
- *Start a food journal so you can keep track of all this information. See page 30 for more tips on how to use a food journal.*
- *If these adjustments don't fix things, cut back to 80 grams of Net Carbs a day.*
- *If that does not help, level down to Atkins 40 (see page 45). You'll still have a full variety of foods to choose from, just in more controlled quantities for slow and steady weight loss.*

Low-Carb Tools You Can Use

Whether you're doing Atkins 20, Atkins 40, or Atkins 100, you can find a variety of free tools on Atkins.com to help you succeed on your low-carb lifestyle:

- **The Atkins app:** *Download this free app and search for foods, track your progress, and plan your meals.*
- **Digital weight loss tracker:** *Count carbs and keep track of your exercise, meals, and progress.*

- **Carb counter:** *See how many Net Carbs are in your favorite foods.*
- **Meal plans and shopping lists:** *In addition to the new meal plans featured in this book, you can find more meal plans and shopping lists here, whether you love to cook or would rather grab and go.*
- **Atkins recipes:** *You'll find more than fifty brand-new low-carb recipes in this book, plus you can browse through more than 1,600 mouthwatering low-carb recipes at Atkins.com.*

GET MOVING

It's a sad but well-known fact: we eat too much and exercise too little. According to a report from the Centers for Disease Control and Prevention's National Center for Health Statistics (NCHS) only 23 percent of American adults meet the recommended exercise guidelines. Studies show that our sedentary lifestyles can be blamed for an increasing incidence of heart disease, obesity, diabetes, osteoporosis, early death, and certain forms of cancer.

Why Exercise Matters

Though exercise is not essential on Atkins, the benefits of moving more far outweigh not moving. Here's why:

- Exercise preserves and builds lean body mass (i.e., muscle).
- Exercise improves your mood and helps decrease depression.
- Exercise helps prevent heart disease, diabetes, metabolic syndrome, and other diseases.
- The more active you are, the more carbs you can consume without gaining weight.

- The more muscle you have compared to fat, the more calories your body burns, even at rest.
- Once your workout is over, your metabolism will continue to burn more calories.

How Much Should I Exercise?

The American Heart Association recommends at least 150 minutes of moderate-intensity physical activity a week. That breaks down to at least 30 minutes per day, five times a week. You can shorten that time by exercising more vigorously: the alternate recommendation is at least 75 minutes of vigorous exercise per week.

Walking is an excellent exercise and a great way to get started. It's a natural, functional movement you can do alone or with anyone (your kids, your family, your coworkers). It puts minimal stress on your joints, you can do it anywhere, and no gym membership or special equipment is required other than a pair of shoes. If you're ready to move past walking, try getting your cardio in with bicycling, running, swimming, a stair stepper or climber, a rowing machine, group classes, water aerobics, tennis, or even gardening or dancing. Finally, you can't go wrong with the powerful combination of cardio exercise and strength-training exercise.

Cardio Exercise

Alternating bursts of cardio with intervals of rest or very-low-intensity cardio has been shown to boost your metabolism, increase your postexercise calorie burn, and improve your fitness level.

Warm up for 2 to 5 minutes, and then try doing 20 to 60 seconds of higher-intensity exercise alternated with 40 to 60 seconds of recovery. Continue this for 15 minutes or more. During the higher-intensity portion of this workout, you should be working hard enough that speaking in full sentences is difficult. Depending on your fitness level, you can walk, jog, run, or bike.

Strength-Training Exercise

Focus on exercises that target each major muscle group. If you're a beginner, start out by using light dumbbells (3 to 5 pounds and 8 to 12 pounds) or a set of resistance bands. As your fitness level improves, you can increase the weight of the dumbbells.

What to Eat Before and After Exercise

First, it's important to understand the role protein and carbs play in exercise:

- **Protein:** Exercise depletes critical amino acids such as glutamine and the three branched-chain amino acids valine, isoleucine, and leucine. Amino acids are the building blocks of protein and are used by your body for making muscles, hormones, neurotransmitters, bones, and all sorts of other important things. The protein you eat replenishes your body's supply of branched-chain amino acids. Think meat, chicken, eggs, fish, or whey protein.
- **Carbohydrates:** Exercise draws upon your body's stores of glycogen, which is the stored form of sugar. Glycogen waits in your liver and your muscles for a signal that sugar is needed to fuel your workout. Your body can hold about 1,800 calories of sugar as glycogen, which is plenty to fuel any workout short of a marathon. Your best choices are slow-burning carbs and low-glycemic fruits such as berries, nuts and seeds, or high-fiber whole grains.

Now that you know the role these important macronutrients play in pre- and postexercise nutrition, here's what to eat.

- **Before you exercise:** Your regularly planned meals and snacks throughout the day should help you stay properly fueled for your workout. Schedule your exercise session so that you have something to eat about an hour beforehand. You should aim to have some protein either before or after your workout in order to help promote recovery. Good preworkout snacks include a low-carb nutrition shake or nutrition bar, a hard-boiled egg or two (or deviled eggs), a serving of almonds or olives, or a ham or turkey roll-up. Cottage cheese or Greek yogurt with some fruit can also help fuel your workout. Be careful not to eat too much fiber immediately before you exercise, as this may lead to an upset stomach.

- **After you exercise:** Plan on eating within thirty minutes after exercise—this is an important window when your body is primed to replenish nutrients, restore fluids, and rebuild muscle. Research shows that your body can use about 15 to 30 grams of protein for muscle building after a meal (depending on your body size), so aim to eat about this much protein during the recovery window. A low-carb nutrition shake is a convenient option, as is any low-carb meal that features a combination of protein, high-fiber carbohydrates, and healthy fats, such as a salad with your choice of chicken, fish, or meat.

Low-Carb Diets and Exercise

Though classic sports nutrition tells us that if you exercise you must eat plenty of carbs, research in the last decade has shown this to be completely untrue. Studies have been done on the effect of low-carb diets on a variety of physical activity. From ultraendurance sports (more on this later) to fitness levels in firefighters, the data show that athletes of many different types not only can function but thrive on a low-carb diet. Two major consistencies have been observed with low-carb diets and exercise:

1. *Athletes on a low-carb diet are able to burn fat at a much higher exercise intensity than those on a high-carb diet. Because their body fat supplies a much larger fuel reserve, this suggests that these athletes can go harder for longer.*
2. *When recreational athletes move to a low-carb approach, they tend to lose body fat, while still maintaining strength and improving their body composition. This translates to a better power-to-weight ratio, which improves performance and is very beneficial when doing body-weight exercises or other types of physically demanding activity that you would see in the military.*

One caveat is that for most people there is a transition period while their body adapts to their new fat-burning metabolism. This usually takes at least a few weeks, so be patient with yourself as you adapt—and know that ultimately you will reap the benefits of being fat adapted.

Drink Up!

Hydration is key before, during, and after workouts. Shoot for eight 8-ounce glasses of water a day, although you may need more depending on how intense and long your exercise session is. Your best bet is to keep a water bottle with you at all times and refill it often!

How to Work In Your Workouts

I get it. Not everyone jumps out of bed every morning beyond excited to go break a sweat. Exercise isn't just about committing to hours at the gym. It's about moving more, more often. Here are some ways to sneak additional activity into your day:

- **Walk to work if you can.** *This is a great way to start your day.*
- **Work out at lunchtime.** *A midday exercise break helps boost your energy and can make you more productive in the afternoon.*
- **Make the most of your screen time.** *Try doing sit-ups or stretching while you watch a favorite show, or download or stream an exercise program you can do in the comfort of your living room.*
- **Work out with a buddy.** *Convince a coworker to walk or work out with you at lunchtime. Scheduling workouts with a buddy also creates a commitment that you'll be more likely to honor.*
- **Wake up and work out.** *As the day goes on, it's easy to let your workout fall to the wayside. Start the day by breaking a sweat, and you're more likely to stick with it.*
- **Make small changes for big results.** *Take the stairs instead of the elevator. Park farther away from your office, or get off a stop or two early if you're using public transportation.*
- **Get your family involved.** *Start a tradition of a family walk after dinner, and set up fun activities on the weekends such as hikes and bike rides.*

Low-Carb Diets and Endurance Athletes

Back in the day, "carb loading" before endurance events was the norm. Think plates of pasta the night before and sugary sports drinks and gels during the race. The reason for this is that when an athlete follows a high-carb diet, he or she is dependent on glucose as the primary fuel for exercise. This storage of sugar in the body as glycogen is limited to about one day, or a couple hours of hard exercise. To keep the carb "fuel" tank full, endurance athletes follow the "carb-loading" approach before and during exercise and events.

But more and more research shows that athletes in sporting events lasting more than a couple hours may benefit from following a low-carb diet. Why? The conventional precompetition meal consisting of high-glycemic carbs will raise your insulin level substantially. This can easily lead to a "crash" in energy right when you need it most. The high level of insulin—plus the demands of the muscle cells—may bring your blood sugar down too low just when you need fuel and energy to keep going. Furthermore, insulin suppresses your body's natural ability to burn fat for fuel, so not only will you have a low blood sugar level, but you can't access your stored fat for energy. But it's possible for endurance athletes to train their bodies to use fat more efficiently. The process of switching to using fat for fuel is called "keto adaptation" or "fat adaptation." By using more fat (and less sugar), the stored glycogen is preserved for later use, enabling the athlete to run longer without fatigue, leaving him or her with more glycogen for when it's needed, such as during a sprint finish.

For this reason, a low-carb diet and low-glycemic meals that promote a steady burning of fat for fuel are exactly what's needed, and many anecdotal reports from endurance athletes, as well as new research, support this strategy.

REAL LIFE ON ATKINS 100

The wonderful thing about Atkins 100 is that no foods are off limits. That being said, here's how to enjoy some of your favorite high-carb foods without going overboard:

- Bread
  - Pair your bread with fat, whether spreading it with a glorious pat

of grass-fed butter or dipping it in high-quality olive oil. The fat will help temper the effect on your blood sugar, as well as satisfy your appetite.

– Make this your only high-glycemic food for the day.

– Allow yourself only one slice.

– Instead of a sandwich with two slices of bread, do an open-face one.

– Slice your bread extra thin.

– Eat only low-carb bread.

• Pasta

– Drizzle your pasta with high-quality olive oil or top with a pat of grass-fed butter.

– Make this your only high-glycemic food for the day.

– Stick with half a serving.

– Eat as a garnish with a plate full of sautéed veggies and chicken.

– Mix with zucchini "noodles" or cauliflower rice.

– Try low-carb pasta.

• Potatoes

– Stick with half a serving.

– Eat as a garnish, not a main dish. You can toss a small serving of roasted potatoes with Foundation Vegetables such as roasted cauliflower, broccoli, or Brussels sprouts.

– Craving mashed potatoes? Add steamed and mashed cauliflower with some heavy cream and grass-fed butter for a delicious flavor bomb.

– You want fries with that? Slice half a potato and mix it with half a sweet potato, zucchini, or radish slices with olive oil and seasoning salt and bake until crispy.

We are only human. If you're going to blow your carb budget, make sure it's worth it! For example, if you can't resist a piece of fresh-from-the-oven crusty French bread from your favorite bakery or a serving of your Italian grandma's homemade pasta, don't! Enjoy the decadent treat, and make sure the rest of your meals and snacks for the day are of the low-glycemic variety.

Swap This for That on Atkins 100

Instead of This	Eat This
Ice cream (not low carb)	Berries in heavy cream or in sour cream with sucralose, low-carb ice cream, or our low-carb homemade ice cream recipes on pages 270 and 279
Salty chips	Nuts, seeds, low-carb chips, or homemade kale or zucchini chips
Sugary soft drinks	Sugar-free beverages, sparkling water with lemon or lime slices, or seltzer water with sugar-free syrup
Mashed potatoes	Mashed cauliflower or turnips with cream and butter
A fruit smoothie	A smoothie made of berries, ice cubes, heavy cream or Greek yogurt, and a packet of Splenda plus, if you like, no-sugar vanilla protein powder
Tortillas	Low-carb tortillas or lettuce leaves
Chocolate	Low-carb chocolate candies

HOW TO EYEBALL PORTION SIZES

Even on Atkins 100, it's important to be able to judge portion sizes, especially for higher-carb foods. While the Acceptable Foods list features serving sizes in 5-gram and 10-gram increments, do you really know what ½ cup looks like if you don't have access to a ½-cup measure? Here's how you can eyeball your portions, even on the go!

Breads, Grains, and Pasta

1 (1-ounce) slice of bread	An index card
1 (2-ounce) piece of Italian bread	A bar of soap
1 (3-ounce) bagel	A can of tuna
½ cup rice, cereal, or pasta	½ baseball
1 (2-ounce) muffin	A cupcake wrapper

Fruits and Vegetables

1 medium fruit or ¾ cup cut-up fruit	A tennis ball
1 cup green salad	A fist
½ cup cooked vegetables	A scoop of ice cream

Protein and Cheese

2 tablespoons peanut butter	Two tea bags
3 ounces beef, chicken, or pork	A small pack of tissues
1 ounce of cheese	A pair of dice
1 ounce of nuts	A Ping-Pong ball

Snacks and Desserts

1 ounce of chips	A medium-size handful
1 (3-inch) piece of cake	A small stack of business cards
1 cup of ice cream	A baseball

Measurements	
1 tablespoon	A tea bag
1 teaspoon	A thimble
1 cup	A fist or a baseball
¼ cup	A large egg

MOVING FORWARD WITH MEAL PLANS AND MORE!

What's next? Keep reading to find out how to shop so you can transform your kitchen and pantry to perfectly fit your low-carb needs. Finally, once that's all dialed in, it's time to explore our satisfying and unique meal plans, featuring some of our brand-new recipes that you can easily customize for Atkins 20, Atkins 40, and Atkins 100.

PART TWO

Putting It All Together: Meal Plans, Low-Carb Hacks, and More

CHAPTER 4

PLANNING, PREP, SHOPPING, AND ATKINS MEAL PLANS

Before anything else, preparation is the key to success.
—*Alexander Graham Bell, American inventor*

IF YOU'RE READY to break free from the sugar- and carb-heavy standard American diet, if you want to start enjoying the increased energy and overall improvement in wellness you'll experience with Atkins 100's delicious and satisfying everyday eating solution, it's time to gather the right foods and meal plans so you have them at your fingertips.

To start, I'll show you some valuable meal-planning and shopping hacks that will make living a low-carb lifestyle a no-brainer, and then I'll follow up with everything you need to get your kitchen into tip-top shape. Finally, you'll be ready to try our Atkins 100 meal plans, which can easily be modified for Atkins 40 and Atkins 20.

HOW TO MEAL PLAN LIKE A PRO

Planning and shopping for meals don't have to be a chore, especially if the outcome is a new, sustainable way of eating. Here are some suggestions:

- **Map out your meals.** Start by using the meal plans on pages 100–107 as your guide. Don't feel pressured to have weeks and weeks of breakfasts, lunches, dinners, and snacks mapped out, because, of course, your plans will change. Think of the week ahead and anticipate what your needs will be.

- **Make a list of go-to meals.** Winging it without a plan during busy weeks can easily result in a last-minute fast-food run. Put together a list of lower-carb versions of go-to meals you can rely on in a pinch that are made from ingredients you usually have on hand, such as tacos, chili, soups, salads, and more.

- **Embrace the recipe search.** Starting on page 181, you'll find more than fifty brand-new delicious low-carb recipes you can add to your recipe collection. But there's no need to stop there; with all the colorful recipes you can find online and in cookbooks, it's easy to become engrossed in the delightful search for new low-carb recipes. You can also find more than fifteen hundred low-carb recipes at Atkins.com. Don't forget to save your faves!

- **Share and share alike.** If you join the Atkins Community at Atkins.com, you'll find plenty of like-minded folks who are passionate about living a low-carb lifestyle and willing to share their favorite low-carb recipes, tips, and tricks.

- **Plan for leftovers.** Leftovers can be a lifesaver during hectic weeks! Package individual servings of leftovers for lunches or make a big pot of chili that can feed your family for a couple of dinners. Tired of eggs? Here's a hack: heat up your dinner leftovers and eat them for breakfast.

Another Reason to Love Leftovers

Typical carb-heavy foods such as pasta, potatoes, and rice can spike your blood sugar in a profound fashion because they contain lots of rapidly digested starch. Therefore, with Atkins 100, we recommend limited servings of these foods. But research shows that if these starches are cooked and then left to cool (leftover rice, anyone?), some of the high-glycemic starch converts into low-glycemic or indigestible resistant starch. This process, known as retrogradation, results in a chemical change to the structure of carbohydrates so that they are much more difficult for the human digestive tract to break down. Often, resistant starches pass into the large intestine, where they have prebiotic benefits and your gut bacteria converts them into short-chain fatty acids, which have a variety of health benefits as described in chapter 1. Because resistant starch is not absorbed by the digestive tract, it also contributes fewer calories to your diet and does not have nearly the same impact on your blood sugar as freshly cooked starch does. Research on resistant starch suggests that the longer a food is cooled, the more resistant starch is formed, so let those leftovers sit for twelve to twenty-four hours (in the fridge, of course). You can reheat your leftovers without destroying the resistant starch as long as you don't heat them above 140°F. It also appears that acid can help the formation of resistant starch, so add some vinegar to your potato or pasta salad or a splash of rice vinegar to your fried rice.

LOW-CARB SHOPPING HACKS

Navigating the grocery store aisles can seem daunting at times, especially when you are faced with an array of healthy and not so healthy choices. Here's what to do:

- **Pick a shopping day and make a shopping list.** Once you have a list of meals you plan to prepare, make a list and check it twice. This chore is easier than ever before with all the grocery shopping apps that let you build your shopping list and share it with your family.

- **Heed the health halo.** Food marketing can be tricky, and the way a food is labeled can imply a benefit when there really is none, known as a "health halo." Foods filled with added sugars, refined carbs, and other unhealthy ingredients may still have labels such as "natural," "light," "organic," "healthy," "gluten free," and so on. So before you chow down on a package of organic or gluten-free cookies, read the label. You may find that they are sky high in naturally occurring and added sugars and have too many carbs for a single serving.

- **Peruse the perimeter.** Your meal mainstays—vegetables, fruits, proteins, and dairy products—live on the perimeter of the grocery store. Healthy protein—chicken, fish, eggs, beef, turkey, pork, and tofu—keeps you fuller for longer, and it helps to preserve fat-burning lean muscle, while fresh produce is packed with nutrients. Use caution when passing through the inner aisles, where the candy, cookies, sugary cereals, and soda live.

- **Go for pickup or delivery.** Many grocery stores and grocery shopping services offer pickup or delivery for a small fee, which means you can build your shopping list online and schedule a time when you'd like to pick up your groceries or have them delivered. This can be a lifesaver if you don't have time to shop and also prevents impulse buying.

- **Eat before you shop.** Make sure you have a low-carb snack before you hit the grocery store so cravings don't strike just as you mistakenly wander into an inner aisle under the pretense of buying more olive oil and emerge with a package of Oreos. The same goes if you are ordering online; though it's much easier to stick to your list, the potential is still there if you are hungry enough!

- **Plan for your sweet tooth.** Have berries on hand when you start craving something sweet, or make one of the low-carb dessert recipes starting on page 265 or on Atkins.com.

Learn to Read a Nutrition Label

Nutrition Facts

1 servings per container
Serving size 1 Shake (325 mL)

Amount per serving
Calories 170

	% Daily Value*
Total Fat 9g	12%
Saturated Fat 2.5g	13%
Trans Fat 0g	
Polyunsaturated Fat 0.5g	
Monounsaturated Fat 6g	
Cholesterol 15mg	5%
Sodium 160mg	7%
Total Carbohydrate 9g	3%
Dietary Fiber 5g	18%
Total Sugars 2g	
Includes 0g Added Sugars	0%
Protein 15g	28%
Vitamin D 0.3mcg	2%
Calcium 240mg	20%
Iron 3mg	15%
Potassium 660mg	15%
Vitamin C 9mg	10%
Niacin 4.5mg	30%
Vitamin B6 0.5mg	30%
Vitamin B12 1.4mcg	60%
Pantothenic Acid 2.5mg	50%

*The % Daily Value (DV) tells you how much a nutrient in a serving of food contributes to a daily diet. 2,000 calories a day is used for general nutrition advice.

- **Serving size:** *The amount shown on the label, as well as calories per serving, refers to a single serving. Beware, because many packages contain more than one serving.*
- **Fat:** *The only fat you need to avoid is trans fat, which has been shown to increase levels of "bad" LDL cholesterol while decreasing levels of "good" HDL cholesterol. Manufacturers are no longer allowed to put trans fats into their products, but don't be fooled by a label that lists 0 grams of trans fat. Because of a labeling loophole, a product can contain up to 0.5 grams of trans*

fat per serving and say it has none. A half gram can add up if you have more than one serving daily. If the ingredients list includes partially hydrogenated oil, hydrogenated oil, or shortening, the product contains trans fat.

- **Total Carbohydrate:** *Remember to subtract grams of dietary fiber from total grams of carbs to get Net Carbs. Some low-sugar packaged foods use sugar alcohols or allulose to replace sugar. These sweeteners don't metabolize as sugar in your body and have very little impact on your blood sugar. In this case, subtract fiber, sugar alcohols, or allulose from total carbs to arrive at the Net Carb count. Don't get confused and subtract grams of sugar; subtract only the sugar alcohol or allulose number.*

- **Total Sugars and Added Sugars:** *Identifying sugar on a nutrition label is becoming easier, because all manufacturers are now required to list grams of added sugars. You can see all the various aliases that added sugars go by on page 18.*

- **% Daily Value:** *The Daily Value (DV) is the recommended amount of each nutrient for average adults and is based on a 2,000-calorie diet. If the DV of a nutrient is 5 percent or less, the food is considered to be low in that nutrient; if it is 20 percent or higher, it is considered high.*

·····························

Tip: *The DV for added sugars is 10 percent of total calories (based on a 2,000-calorie diet). If you do the math, that's 200 calories, which is equal to 50 grams of sugar, which is not compatible with Atkins 100.*

·····························

- **Ingredients:** *This includes everything in the food product from highest to lowest content. This is where you'll find added sugars and trans fats, as well as naturally occurring sugars and whole* *grains. If you see the word "enriched" before a grain, it means the grain has been stripped of the germ and bran and fortified with nutrients.*

Watch Out for Whole Wheat

If you see "whole wheat" on a label, it can have just as big a glycemic impact as white bread. Go for breads made with sprouted grains, which are grains such as wheat berry or soy that are soaked in water until they sprout, or ancient grains, which are technically not grains but actually seeds or plants that have been cultivated for centuries, such as amaranth, barley, and farro. Breads made from these grains tend to be lower in carbs and less processed.

CURATING A LOW-CARB KITCHEN

To curate means to choose something carefully and thoughtfully organize or present it. This is my goal for you: a carefully curated low-carb kitchen.

Once your kitchen is organized (who knows, maybe you'll even be motivated to alphabetize your spice rack!), I'll show you how to stock it with delicious low-carb staples, which makes it easy to plan and shop for meals, as well as integrate different ingredients as you add new low-carb recipes to your weekly menu. Though no food is forbidden on Atkins 100, this guide should help you make the best choices.

First, it's time to give your kitchen some love. Follow these tips for what to toss and what to keep in your fridge, freezer, and pantry. Don't forget to wipe down shelves and clean as you go.

FRIDGE

TOSS:

- Anything that is expired and anything that doesn't look or smell good, such as vegetables past their prime.
- Anything containing more than 5 grams of sugar and more than 15 grams of Net Carbs per serving. Read the labels on the other packaged foods in your fridge, such as barbecue sauce, salad dressing, low-fat and sweetened yogurt, spaghetti sauce, jams and jellies, and so on. You can keep items that are lower in sugar and Net Carbs per serving.

KEEP:

- Most vegetables and some fruits (see Appendix D for a list of vegetables and fruits you can keep in your fridge).
- Meats, eggs, dairy products, and oils.
- Condiments such as salsa, hot sauce, mustard, honey mustard, low-sugar or sugar-free salad dressings, mayonnaise, horseradish, pesto, lemon or lime juice, and soy sauce or tamari.

FREEZER

TOSS:

- Anything that's expired or freezer burned.
- Although they are popular with kids and adults alike, processed foods such as waffles, breakfast pastries, pizza, pasta, chicken nuggets, and ice cream are high in sugar and Net Carbs. Once again, make sure anything you keep has fewer than 5 grams of sugar and fewer than 15 grams of Net Carbs.

KEEP:

- Frozen broccoli, cauliflower, bell pepper, and spinach.

- Frozen vegetables such as corn and potatoes; they are higher in carbs but can still be a part of your Atkins 100 lifestyle.
- Frozen berries and other fruits.
- Protein such as frozen meats, shrimp, seafood, and others.

Thumbs-up for Frozen Food

For some reason, there is a perception that fresh fruits and vegetables are nutritionally superior to frozen. However, there is some research that suggests that the nutrient content in fresh produce declines over time. Certain antioxidants and vitamins slowly degrade, and the days or weeks that it takes to transport produce across the country and then sit in the grocery store before you buy it can result in a significant change to the nutrient content. One study found that vitamin C losses in vegetables stored at 39°F were between 15 and 77 percent, though they depended on the type of vegetable analyzed. This doesn't mean that we shouldn't eat fresh fruits and veggies, but since vegetables are frozen almost immediately after they've been harvested, the nutrient content does not decline as dramatically—and frozen fruits and vegetables tend to be more affordable!

Tip: See Appendix D for a full list of vegetables and fruits that you may find in the frozen section that are great to have on hand in your freezer.

PANTRY

TOSS:

- Most canned soups are high in carbs; read the labels, and toss anything that contains more than 5 grams of sugar or 15 grams of Net Carbs per serving.

- Canned fruit packed with added sugar and syrup.
- Breakfast cereals, crackers, chips, cookies, and more.
- Instant oatmeal unless it has fewer than 5 grams of sugar and 15 grams of Net Carbs per serving.
- Spices that smell stale or are years old.

KEEP:

- High-fiber bran or flax cereal with 15 grams of Net Carbs or less.
- Cheese chips, flax chips, snap pea chips, and high-fiber seed crackers with 15 grams Net Carbs or fewer.
- Canned tomato, chicken, vegetable, broccoli, and vegetable cream soups and butternut squash soup.
- Canned fruit in its own juice (just drain the juice before eating).
- Canned fish and seafood such as tuna, salmon, sardines, and anchovies.
- Canned tomatoes, tomato paste, and pasta or tomato sauce without added sugar or with 5 grams of sugar or less per serving.
- Canned beans (though higher in carbs, they can be part of your Atkins 100 lifestyle).
- Salsas.
- Bottled hot sauces.
- Canned green chilies.
- Canned pumpkin.
- Chicken, beef, and vegetable stock or broth.
- Chicken, beef, and vegetable bouillon.
- Nuts and seeds.
- Roasted red peppers (rinse before using if there is sugar in the ingredients).
- Sun-dried tomatoes in oil.
- Artichoke hearts.

- Capers.
- Pesto and other vegetable-based sauces.
- Other canned low-carb vegetables.
- Dill pickles.
- Italian-style pickled vegetables.
- Nut butters.
- Tahini.
- Olives.
- Herbs and spices.
- Tea.
- Coffee.
- Cider and wine vinegar.
- Balsamic vinegar (check label for sugar content).
- Rice wine vinegar (check label for sugar content).
- Worcestershire sauce (check label for sugar content).
- Cooking oils, such as canola oil, olive oil, and coconut oil (see "Healthy Cooking Oils," page 92).

....

Tip: Keep a well-stocked pantry. It's not fun when you run out of a crucial ingredient you need for a recipe when you're in the midst of cooking, and many of the items in your pantry are nonperishable and should last for some time. You can use the above list not only as a guide for what to keep in your pantry if you already have it but as suggestions for what to add.

....

Waste Not, Want Not

Please do not waste food! You can donate nonperishable food that you'd rather not keep to your local food bank.

Healthy Cooking Oils

Healthy cooking oils are a great source of healthy fats and fat-soluble vitamins and a pantry essential. Here is a list of oils you can use to sauté, bake, stir-fry, or drizzle:

- **Avocado oil:** *This oil is unrefined like extra-virgin olive oil, but has a higher smoke point, which makes it a great choice for stir-fries. It contains both monounsaturated and polyunsaturated fats, as well as vitamin E.*
- **Canola oil:** *Made from the seeds of the rapeseed plant, canola oil is one of the healthiest cooking oils, as it contains a higher amount of omega-3 fats than most other oils, which lower blood pressure and heart rate. It has a high smoke point and is great for sautéing, baking, and marinating. Look for cold-pressed or unprocessed canola oil, if available.*
- **Coconut oil:** *Coconut oil is rich in saturated fats. It also helps control blood sugar and facilitates the absorption of calcium. With a subtle coconut flavor, this oil makes a great substitute for butter when baking.*
- **Flaxseed oil:** *Flaxseed oil is high in omega-3s and has a very low smoke point, so it's not good for cooking, but you can use it to make a salad dressing or add some to your smoothie.*
- **Grape seed oil:** *As the name suggests, grape seed oil is extracted from the seeds of grapes. It's high in polyunsaturated fats and vitamin E. It also has a high smoke point, so it's great for sautéing, stir-frying, and roasting.*
- **Olive oil:** *One of the most popular cooking oils, olive oil is a staple in many households. Opt for extra-virgin olive oil, which is made from the first pressing of olives. Extra-virgin olive oil is high in antioxidants called polyphenols, which provide heart-healthy benefits. It has a lower smoke point compared to other oils, so it's*

best for low- to medium-heat cooking. Use olive oil to sauté vegeta-bles or combine with balsamic vinegar for an easy salad dressing.

- **Peanut oil:** *Made from unshelled peanuts, peanut oil contains heart-healthy phytosterols, plant fats associated with lower cho-lesterol and cancer prevention. Peanut oil is flavorful with a nutty taste and smell, and is well suited for deep frying, as well as roasting and sautéing, thanks to its high smoke point.*

- **Sesame oil:** *Sesame oil is very flavorful and contains both mono-unsaturated and polyunsaturated fats. It has a high smoke point, so it's good for cooking, and it especially goes well in Asian recipes.*

- **Walnut oil:** *This oil has a good ratio of omega-6 to omega-3 fatty acids, which helps control inflammation. It has a low smoke point, so it's not good for cooking, but you can drizzle it over fruit or add it to a coffee drink.*

LET'S START SHOPPING!

Now that your kitchen is carefully curated, there's a delicious world of low-carb living waiting for you. I've put together a suggested shopping list with many options to choose from, and you may have discovered as you organized your fridge, freezer, and pantry that you already have a lot of these foods on hand.

Produce

This list includes colorful vegetables and plenty of other essentials for salads, snacks, side dishes, and more. You should consume a minimum of 12 to 15 grams of Net Carbs of Foundation Vegetables a day, which is about 6 cups of raw vegetables or 2 cups of cooked veggies, but you can mix and match them to suit your needs. You'll also see that I've included starchy vegeta-bles, which are higher in Net Carbs. The Net Carbs of these vegetables range from 0 grams to a little more than 5 grams of Net Carbs per serving, and this list is organized from the smallest amount of Net Carbs to the greatest. Next is a list of fruits, organized in the same way. For more details on specific Net Carb counts and serving sizes of each food, see Appendix D.

FOUNDATION VEGETABLES

- Sprouts
- Chicory greens
- Endive
- Olives, green or black
- Watercress
- Arugula
- Radishes
- Spinach
- Bok choy
- Lettuce, all types
- Turnip greens
- Hearts of palm
- Radicchio
- Mushrooms
- Artichokes
- Celery
- Pickles, dill
- Broccoli rabe
- Broccoli
- Sauerkraut
- Avocados
- Daikon radishes
- Onions, red or white
- Zucchini
- Cucumbers
- Cauliflower
- Beet greens
- Fennel
- Okra
- Rhubarb
- Swiss chard
- Asparagus
- Broccolini
- Bell peppers
- Eggplants
- Kale
- Scallions
- Turnips
- Tomatoes
- Jicama
- Yellow squash
- Cabbage
- Green beans
- Leeks
- Shallots
- Brussels sprouts
- Spaghetti squash
- Kohlrabi
- Pumpkin
- Garlic
- Snow peas
- Tomatoes

STARCHY VEGETABLES

- Carrots
- Butternut squash
- Rutabagas
- Acorn squash
- Beets
- Corn
- Parsnips
- Peas
- Sweet potatoes
- Potatoes

FRUITS

- Rhubarb
- Coconuts
- Blackberries
- Boysenberries
- Raspberries
- Cranberries
- Cantaloupes
- Strawberries
- Watermelons
- Gooseberries
- Guava
- Grapefruit
- Honeydew melons
- Lemon juice
- Lime juice
- Blueberries
- Figs
- Apples
- Plums
- Clementines
- Oranges
- Peaches
- Kiwis
- Pears
- Pineapples
- Mangoes
- Cherries
- Bananas
- Grapes
- Dates
- Raisins

Tip: Prep food in advance. Wash and dry salad greens and cut up veggies so everything is ready to grab and go when you're throwing together meals or need a quick snack. There's nothing worse than discovering a forgotten piece of fruit way past its prime hiding behind an expired jar of mustard in a dark corner of your fridge!

NUTS AND SEEDS AND THEIR BUTTERS

- Almonds
- Almond butter
- Brazil nuts
- Cashews
- Cashew butter
- Coconut
- Hazelnuts
- Macadamia nuts
- Macadamia butter
- Peanuts
- Peanut butter
- Pecans
- Pine nuts
- Pistachios
- Pumpkin seeds
- Sesame seeds
- Soy "nut" butter
- Sunflower seeds
- Sunflower seed butter
- Tahini
- Walnuts

WHOLE GRAINS

- Barley
- Brown rice
- Coconut flour
- Couscous
- Grits
- Millet
- Oat bran
- Oatmeal, steel cut
- Polenta
- Quinoa
- Wheat bran
- Wheat germ
- Whole wheat pasta
- Whole wheat bread

LEGUMES

- Black beans
- Cannellini beans
- Chickpeas
- Edamame
- Hummus
- Kidney beans
- Split peas

. . . .

Tip: *See Appendix D for serving sizes and Net Carbs*
for whole grains and legumes.

. . . .

MEAT

- Beef
- Ham
- Lamb
- Pork
- Veal
- Venison

FOWL

- Chicken
- Cornish hen
- Duck
- Goose
- Pheasant
- Quail
- Turkey

....

Tip: Avoid chicken nuggets, breaded cutlets, and anything that has been deep fried, stuffed, breaded, battered, or coated in flour.

....

FISH

- Cod
- Flounder
- Halibut
- Herring
- Salmon
- Sardines
- Sole
- Tuna
- Trout

SHELLFISH

- Clams
- Crabmeat
- Lobster
- Mussels*
- Oysters*
- Shrimp
- Squid

Mussels and oysters are slightly higher in Net Carbs.

DAIRY PRODUCTS

- Cottage cheese, full fat
- Eggs
- Half-and-half
- Heavy cream
- Light cream
- Mayonnaise

- Plain coconut milk
- Sour cream, full fat
- Unsweetened almond milk
- Unsweetened soymilk
- Unsweetened yogurt, full fat

....

Tip: *You can use liquid cream or half-and-half in your coffee.*
Watch out for packaged creamers; many are full of sugar,
high-fructose corn syrup, or maltodextrin, a high-carb starch.

....

CHEESE

- Bleu cheese
- Cheddar or Colby
- Cream cheese, full fat
- Feta
- Goat
- Gouda
- Havarti
- Jarlsberg
- Laughing Cow
- Mozzarella, whole milk
- Parmesan
- Romano
- String
- Swiss

FATS AND OILS

- Butter
- Mayonnaise (watch out for added sugar)
- Oils (see "Healthy Cooking Oils" on page 92 for examples)

BEVERAGES

- Clear broth/bouillon
- Club soda
- Decaffeinated or regular coffee and tea, sugar-free iced tea
- Diet soda
- Herb tea without added sugar
- No-calorie flavored seltzer
- Unflavored soy/almond milk
- Water, including:
  – Filtered
  – Mineral
  – Spring
  – Tap

....
Tip: *Always check the Nutrition Label for the sugar content. You can pump up the flavor of your water with a few squeezes of lemon or lime.*
....

HERBS AND SPICES

- Basil
- Black pepper
- Cayenne pepper
- Chives, fresh or dehydrated
- Cilantro
- Dill
- Garlic
- Ginger, fresh
- Oregano
- Parsley
- Rosemary, dried
- Sage, ground
- Salt
- Tarragon

....
Tip: *If you need to restock your spice rack, this list is a great place to start, but your options are endless. Just watch for spice mixes that contain added sugar.*
....

SALAD DRESSINGS

- Balsamic vinegar
- Blue cheese dressing
- Caesar dressing
- Italian dressing
- Lemon juice
- Lime juice
- Ranch dressing
- Red wine vinegar

NONCALORIC SWEETENERS*

- Erythritol-stevia blend (Truvia)
- Saccharin
- Stevia (SugarLeaf)
- Sucralose (Splenda)
- Xylitol

*Count each packet as 1 gram of Net Carbs.

MOVING ON TO ATKINS 100 MEAL PLANS

These meal plans emphasize healthy choices and showcase the wide variety of food you can eat on Atkins 100, as well as some of our delicious new low-carb recipes featured in this book and some favorite low-carb recipes from Atkins.com. Though you can follow these meal plans to the letter, you can also make your own substitutions based on your personal tastes and budget, the seasonality of produce, and what you have on hand in your fridge, freezer, and pantry. You can use the Acceptable Foods list on page 303 and the Atkins app to check if your substitutions measure up. You don't need to stick with these meal plans in the order they are listed, and you can swap breakfasts, lunches, and dinners with other meals with comparable Net Carb counts. What is also so great about these meals plans is that you can level down to Atkins 40 or Atkins 20.

ATKINS 100, ATKINS 40, AND ATKINS 20 MEAL PLANS

Bold and Italic: recipe found in this book; _italic and underlined_: recipe found on the Atkins website.

DAY 1

	ATKINS 100	ATKINS 40	ATKINS 20
Breakfast	**Broccolini and Bacon Egg Bites (page 198)** 1 slice Ezekiel bread *Net Carbs: 22 g; FV: 1	**Broccolini and Bacon Egg Bites** ¼ cup fresh blueberries Net Carbs: 9 g; FV: 1	**Broccolini and Bacon Egg Bites** Net Carbs: 4 g; FV: 1
Snack	**Chili-Spiced Papaya (page 259)** 12 roasted almonds Net Carbs: 11 g; FV: 0	½ pear 12 roasted almonds Net Carbs: 11 g; FV: 0	½ avocado ¼ teaspoon Mexican Tajin seasoning Net Carbs: 1 g; FV: 1

Lunch	*Moroccan Chicken Mason Jar Salad (page 209)* ⅓ cup cooked quinoa Net Carbs: 15 g; FV: 3	*Moroccan Chicken Mason Jar Salad* 2 tablespoons sliced almonds Net Carbs: 6 g; FV: 3	*Moroccan Chicken Mason Jar Salad* Net Carbs: 5 g; FV: 3
Snack	13 grape tomatoes 12 herb seed crackers ¼ cup hummus Net Carbs: 33 g; FV: 6	*Dukkah "Deviled" Eggs (page 254)* Net Carbs: 1 g; FV: 0	25 green olives 1 ounce Havarti cheese Net Carbs: 0 g; FV: 0
Dinner	*Lemon Baked Cod with Braised Cauliflower and Greens (page 243)* ⅓ cup cooked quinoa Net Carbs: 20 g; FV: 7	*Lemon Baked Cod with Braised Cauliflower and Greens* ¼ cup mashed cooked turnips Net Carbs: 11 g; FV: 9	*Lemon Baked Cod with Braised Cauliflower and Greens* Net Carbs: 9 g; FV: 7
TOTALS	Carbs: 131 g; Net Carbs: 101 g; Protein: 105 g; Fiber: 30 g; Fat: 103 g; Calories: 1,848; FV: 17	Carbs: 57 g; Net Carbs: 38 g; Protein: 94 g; Fiber: 19 g; Fat: 108 g; Calories: 1,551; FV: 13	Carbs: 38 g; Net Carbs: 19 g; Protein: 89 g; Fiber: 18 g; Fat: 112 g; Calories: 1,502; FV: 12

DAY 2

Breakfast	*Smoked Salmon Stack (page 187)* 1 slice Ezekiel bread Net Carbs: 17 g; FV: 2	*Smoked Salmon Stack* 1 slice *Sweet Potato Toast (page 188)* Net Carbs: 10 g; FV: 2	*Smoked Salmon Stack* Net Carbs: 5 g; FV: 2
Snack	1 medium pear 2 tablespoons peanut butter Net Carbs: 25 g; FV: 0	10 black olives 1 marinated artichoke heart Net Carbs: 2 g; FV: 2	*Cheesy Cauliflower Bites (page 249)* Net Carbs: 5 g; FV: 2

Lunch	Spinach, Asparagus, and Charred Scallion Frittata (page 211) 1 slice Ezekiel bread Net Carbs: 18 g; FV: 3	Spinach, Asparagus, and Charred Scallion Frittata ¼ cup fresh blueberries Net Carbs: 10 g; FV: 3	Spinach, Asparagus, and Charred Scallion Frittata Net Carbs: 6 g; FV: 3
Snack	Sweet Potato Toast (page 188) 2 tablespoons black bean dip ¼ avocado Net Carbs: 9 g; FV: 5	1 avocado ¼ teaspoon Mexican Tajin seasoning Net Carbs: 3 g; FV: 3	1 avocado blended with 3 tablespoons mayonnaise 5 radishes Net Carbs: 3 g; FV: 3
Dinner	Prosciutto Chicken with Lots of Greens (page 229) ⅓ cup prepared polenta Net Carbs: 18 g; FV: 3	Prosciutto Chicken with Lots of Greens 2 tablespoons prepared polenta Net Carbs: 9 g; FV: 3	Prosciutto Chicken with Lots of Greens Net Carbs: 3 g; FV: 3
Dessert	Fresh Peach and Cinnamon No-Churn Ice Cream (page 279) Net Carbs: 10 g; FV: 0	No-Churn Mint Chip Ice Cream (page 270) Net Carbs: 8 g; FV:0	
TOTALS	Carbs: 123 g; Net Carbs: 97 g; Protein: 111 g; Fiber: 27 g; Fat: 103 g; Calories: 1,838; FV: 14	Carbs: 64 g; Net Carbs: 42 g; Protein: 96 g; Fiber: 23 g; Fat: 120 g; Calories: 1,681; FV: 13	Carbs: 40 g; Net Carbs: 22 g; Protein: 97 g; Fiber: 18 g; Fat: 106 g; Calories: 1,487; FV: 14

DAY 3

Breakfast	Warm Escarole with Eggs and Prosciutto (page 200) 3 ounces baked sweet potato Net Carbs: 17 g; FV: 0	Warm Escarole with Eggs and Prosciutto 2 ounces baked sweet potato Net Carbs: 12 g; FV: 0	Warm Escarole with Eggs and Prosciutto Net Carbs: 2 g; FV: 0

Snack	½ medium cucumber ¼ cup hummus *Net Carbs: 14 g; FV: 5*	2 stalks celery 2 tablespoons almond butter *Net Carbs: 5 g; FV: 2*	2 stalks celery ½ cup sliced red pepper 2 tablespoons *Ranch Dressing* *Net Carbs: 5 g; FV: 4*
Lunch	***Red Curry Tofu and Rainbow Chard Stew (page 205)*** 3 tablespoons cooked chickpeas *Net Carbs: 14 g; FV: 4*	***Red Curry Tofu and Rainbow Chard Stew*** 1 tablespoon cooked chickpeas *Net Carbs: 9 g; FV: 4*	***Red Curry Tofu and Rainbow Chard Stew*** *Net Carbs: 8 g; FV: 4*
Snack	***Baked Brie with Warm Grapes and Thyme (page 260)*** 1 cup red grapes *Net Carbs 38 g; FV: 0*	***Mezze Plate with Falafel-Spiced Yogurt Dip (page 256)*** *Net Carbs: 4 g; FV: 2*	***Green Goddess Guacamole with Crunchy Veggies (page 253)*** *Net Carbs: 5 g; FV: 4*
Dinner	***Paprika Pork Chops with Sauerkraut and Mustard (page 233)*** ***Sautéed Apples and Thyme (page 236)*** 1½ cups steamed broccoli *Net Carbs: 15 g; FV: 6*	***Paprika Pork Chops with Sauerkraut and Mustard*** 1 serving ***Cauliflower-Sour Cream Mash (page 235)*** *Net Carbs: 11 g; FV: 5*	***Paprika Pork Chops with Sauerkraut and Mustard*** *Net Carbs: 1 g; FV: 1*
TOTALS	Carbs: 127 g; Net Carbs: 98 g; Protein: 113 g; Fiber: 28 g; Fat: 95 g; Calories: 1,800; FV: 15	Carbs: 62 g; Net Carbs: 41 g; Protein: 109 g; Fiber: 20 g; Fat: 119 g; Calories: 1,754; FV: 14	Carbs: 39 g; Net Carbs: 21 g; Protein: 94 g; Fiber: 19 g; Fat: 100 g; Calories: 1,441; FV: 13

DAY 4

Breakfast	***Green Shakshuka (page 182)*** ½ cup cooked quinoa *Net Carbs: 25 g; FV: 5*	***Green Shakshuka*** 1 serving ***Cauliflower Rice with Butter and Chives (page 183)*** *Net Carbs: 11 g; FV: 7*	***Green Shakshuka*** *Net Carbs: 8 g; FV: 5*

Snack	1 medium pear 1 ounce cheddar cheese *Net Carbs: 21 g; FV: 0*	½ cup blueberries 1 tablespoon sour cream *Net Carbs: 9 g; FV: 0*	*Muffin in a Minute* *Net Carbs: 2 g; FV: 0*
Lunch	**Mediterranean Tuna** **Salad (page 204)** 1 slice Ezekiel bread *Net Carbs: 18 g; FV: 3*	**Mediterranean** **Tuna Salad** 1 low-carb tortilla *Net Carbs: 10 g; FV: 3*	**Mediterranean** **Tuna Salad** *Net Carbs: 6 g; FV: 3*
Snack	½ cup sliced cucumber ½ cup sliced red pepper ¼ cup hummus *Net Carbs: 13 g; FV: 4*	½ cup sliced cucumber ½ cup sliced red pepper *Net Carbs: 4 g; FV: 4*	7 cherry tomatoes *Net Carbs: 3 g; FV: 3*
Dinner	**Crispy Cajun Chicken** **Thighs with Celery** **Ranch Salad (page** **231)** 1 serving **Sweet Potato** **Fries (page 233)** *Net Carbs: 23 g; FV: 1*	**Crispy Cajun Chicken** **Thighs with Celery** **Ranch Salad** ½ cup chopped raw carrots added to the salad *Net Carbs: 8 g; FV: 1*	**Crispy Cajun Chicken** **Thighs with Celery** **Ranch Salad** *Net Carbs: 4 g; FV: 1*
TOTALS	Carbs: 128 g; Net Carbs: 100 g; Protein: 138 g; Fiber: 27 g; Fat: 133 g; Calories: 2,227; FV: 13	Carbs: 72 g; Net Carbs g: 42; Protein: 126 g; Fiber: 31 g; Fat: 123 g; Calories: 1,815; FV: 15	Carbs: 49 g; Net Carbs: 23 g; Protein: 128 g; Fiber: 19 g; Fat: 135 g; Calories: 1,877; FV: 12

DAY 5

Breakfast	**Spicy Sausage Patties** **with Cauliflower Hash** **Browns (page 191)** 1 slice Ezekiel bread *Net Carbs: 17 g; FV: 3*	**Spicy Sausage Patties** **with Cauliflower Hash** **Browns** ½ slice Ezekiel bread *Net Carbs: 11 g; FV: 3*	**Spicy Sausage Patties** **with Cauliflower Hash** **Browns** *Net Carbs: 5 g; FV: 3*

Snack	½ cup plain unsweetened yogurt 1 cup cubed cantaloupe *Net Carbs: 17 g; FV: 0*	½ cup raspberries 12 roasted almonds *Net Carbs: 4 g; FV: 0*	5 radishes 1 tablespoon whipped butter with sea salt *Net Carbs: 1 g; FV: 1*
Lunch	***Vietnamese Shrimp and Vegetable Noodle Bowls (page 221)*** ¾ cup cooked rice noodles *Net Carbs: 41 g; FV: 4*	***Vietnamese Shrimp and Vegetable Noodle Bowls*** 2 tablespoons chopped salted peanuts *Net Carbs: 10 g; FV: 4*	***Vietnamese Shrimp and Vegetable Noodle Bowls*** *Net Carbs: 8 g; FV: 4*
Snack	10 black olives 2 marinated artichoke hearts 1 ounce fresh mozzarella *Net Carbs: 3 g; FV: 3*	10 black olives 2 marinated artichoke hearts 1 ounce fresh mozzarella *Net Carbs: 3 g; FV: 3*	10 black olives 1 ounce Havarti cheese *Net Carbs: 1 g; FV: 1*
Dinner	***"Nachos" Stuffed Chicken Breast (page 236)*** ½ cup refried black beans ½ cup sliced bell pepper ½ avocado *Net Carbs: 20 g; FV: 4*	***"Nachos" Stuffed Chicken Breast*** 2 tablespoons refried black beans ½ cup sliced bell pepper ½ avocado *Net Carbs: 10 g; FV: 4*	***"Nachos" Stuffed Chicken Breast*** 1 avocado *Net Carbs: 6 g; FV: 4*
TOTALS	Carbs: 126 g; Net Carbs: 98 g; Protein: 136 g; Fiber: 27 g; Fat: 114 g; Calories: 2,026; FV: 15	Carbs: 65 g; Net Carbs: 38 g; Protein: 131 g; Fiber g: 26; Fat: 127 g; Calories: 1,866; FV: 15	Carbs: 41 g; Net Carbs: 21 g; Protein: 118 g; Fiber: 19 g; Fat: 128 g; Calories: 1,762; FV: 13

DAY 6

Breakfast	***Hearty Greens and Mushroom Breakfast Scramble (page 185)*** 1 Siete almond flour grain-free tortilla *Net Carbs: 15 g; FV: 4*	***Hearty Greens and Mushroom Breakfast Scramble*** 1 low-carb tortilla *Net Carbs: 11 g; FV: 4*	***Hearty Greens and Mushroom Breakfast Scramble*** *Net Carbs: 7 g; FV: 4*

Snack	15 cherry tomatoes 12 herb seed crackers (Mary's Gone Crackers brand) ¼ cup black bean dip *Net Carbs: 32 g; FV: 7*	½ cup sliced cucumber 5 cherry tomatoes 2 tablespoons black bean dip *Net Carbs: 8 g; FV: 4*	1 avocado *Net Carbs: 3 g; FV: 3*
Lunch	***Tuscan Seared Steak and Shredded Kale Salad (page 217)*** ½ fresh pear *Net Carbs: 16 g; FV: 4*	***Tuscan Seared Steak and Shredded Kale Salad*** ¼ fresh apple *Net Carbs: 10 g; FV: 4*	***Tuscan Seared Steak and Shredded Kale Salad*** *Net Carbs: 5 g; FV: 4*
Snack	1 medium apple 12 roasted almonds *Net Carbs: 22 g; FV: 0*	1 small plum *Net Carbs: 7 g; FV: 0*	5 black olives *Net Carbs: 1 g; FV: 1*
Dinner	***Roasted Salmon with Crushed Green Olive, Lemon, and Fennel Salad (page 226)*** ½ cup steamed parsnips *Net Carbs: 15 g; FV: 13*	***Roasted Salmon with Crushed Green Olive, Lemon, and Fennel Salad*** 2 tablespoons chopped toasted walnuts *Net Carbs: 6 g; FV: 2*	***Roasted Salmon with Crushed Green Olive, Lemon, and Fennel Salad*** *Net Carbs: 5 g; FV: 2*
TOTALS	Carbs: 131 g; Net Carbs: 100 g; Protein: 133 g; Fiber: 31 g; Fat: 123 g; Calories: 2,130; FV: 27	Carbs: 71 g; Net Carbs: 42 g; Protein: 125 g; Fiber: 29 g; Fat: 117 g; Calories: 1,762; FV: 14	Carbs: 40 g; Net Carbs: 21 g; Protein: 117 g; Fiber: 19 g; Fat: 126 g; Calories: 1,734; FV: 13

DAY 7

Breakfast	***"Zucchini Bread" Protein Pancakes (page 196)*** ½ baked apple *Net Carbs: 17 g; FV: 1*	***"Zucchini Bread" Protein Pancakes*** ¼ cup fresh blueberries *Net Carbs: 12 g; FV: 1*	***"Zucchini Bread" Protein Pancakes*** *Net Carbs: 7 g; FV: 1*

Snack	**6 Peach Caprese Skewers (page 262)** 1 cup grapes Net Carbs: 29 g; FV: 1	½ cup sliced fresh strawberries Net Carbs: 5 g; FV: 0	6 radishes 20 green olives Net Carbs: 1 g; FV: 1
Lunch	**Muffaletta "Hero" (page 215)** 1 slice Ezekiel bread Net Carbs: 18 g; FV: 5	**Muffaletta "Hero"** 1 low-carb tortilla Net Carbs: 10 g; FV: 5	**Muffaletta "Hero"** Net Carbs: 6 g; FV: 5
Snack	¾ cup sliced cucumber ½ cup sliced red pepper 1 tablespoon bottled ranch dressing Net Carbs: 5 g; FV: 4	⅓ medium cucumber 5 black olives 2 pieces marinated artichoke heart Net Carbs: 6 g; FV:6	**Zucchini Fritters with Sun-dried Tomato Pesto (page 251)** Net Carbs: 5 g; FV: 4
Dinner	**Seared Hanger Steak with Harissa Butter and Spinach (page 241)** ½ cup cannellini beans Net Carbs: 14 g; FV: 1	**Seared Hanger Steak with Harissa Butter and Spinach** ¼ cup cannellini beans Net Carbs: 9 g; FV: 1	**Seared Hanger Steak with Harissa Butter and Spinach** Net Carbs: 3 g; FV: 1
TOTALS	Carbs: 117 g; Net Carbs: 83 g; Protein: 156 g; Fiber: 32 g; Fat: 127 g; Calories: 2,167; FV: 12	Carbs: 79 g; Net Carbs: 42 g; Protein: 146 g; Fiber: 38 g; Fat: 115 g; Calories: 1,828; FV: 13	Carbs: 40 g; Net Carbs: 22 g; Protein: 146 g; Fiber: 17 g; Fat: 142 g; Calories: 1,976; FV: 12

*Numbers are rounded.

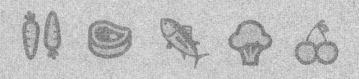

CHAPTER 5

LOW-CARB COOKING HACKS

No one is born a great cook, one learns by doing.
—*Julia Child*

NOW THAT YOUR KITCHEN is curated and stocked with delicious low-carb foods, and you have an array of meal plans and recipes to choose from, I'll show you my favorite hacks for low-carb cooking to add flavor and variety to your meals and snacks, plus cooking techniques every home cook should have under their apron, because cooking on Atkins 100 isn't much different from "regular" cooking, other than limiting certain ingredients, such as sugar and refined grains. And guess what? The whole family can do Atkins 100, especially with my family-friendly cooking tips.

WHAT'S YOUR COOKING STYLE?

Regardless of your attitude toward cooking, keep reading to find out what your cooking style is and how to make the most of it on Atkins 100. Following are some recommendations based on your comfort level in the kitchen; whether you're a bake sale master or use your oven for extra storage, Atkins 100 is doable for anybody!

Are You "by the (Cook)book"?

You probably thrive on a structured routine, with easy breakfasts, lunches, dinners, and snacks you can prepare and eat without having to think too much about them. You make the most of leftovers, and you are content with rotating through a few reliable recipes. If this is you, I've made things supereasy: just stick with the Atkins 100 shopping list, meal plans, and Acceptable Foods list.

Are You a "No-Cook" Cook?
Is your cooking style more of the "no-cook" style? See page 129 for my favorite hacks for eating out on Atkins 100.

Would You Rather Wing It?

You get bored quickly, and variety is key for you! You love exploring Pinterest and Instagram for new recipes and inspiration, and you are quite confident adding your personal touch to any meal. You know how to make substitutions on the fly and gladly take on the challenge of creating new meals based on ingredients you have on hand, but you're also passionate about perusing the produce aisle or farmer's market for vegetables and herbs in season. If this is you, you may have already taken a sneak peek at the low-carb recipes in this book and are ready to start cooking. You can use the Atkins 100 meal plans for more inspiration. Feel free to mix and match meals and recipes to give you the variety you crave.

Are You a Little of Both?

You thrive on a steady repertoire of go-to breakfasts, lunches, and dinners, but when given the chance, you love to don your apron and mix it up with new recipes and different ingredients. Use the Atkins 100 meal plans as your general guide and choose a few new low-carb recipes each week to spice up your routine.

THE SECRETS OF LOW-CARB COOKING

Even if you're a klutz in the kitchen, you can elevate your low-carb cooking game with the following simple recipes and essential cooking techniques.

MARINADES AND MORE

Many store-bought spice mixes, marinades, and sauces are sneaky sources of sugar. When you make your own, you can control the ingredients while adding lots of flavor:

- Spice rubs are dry mixtures—including salt, pepper, dried herbs and spices such as paprika, rosemary, thyme, cumin, cayenne, chili and chipotle pepper, and garlic and onion powder—that are rubbed onto fish, poultry, or meat. The rub penetrates only the surface of the meat, creating an outside "crust" that provides a spicy, flavorful kick.
- Marinades are mixtures of acidic juices with oils, herbs, and/or spices that are used to flavor and tenderize food, usually in the fridge, for as little as thirty minutes to hours or days. Marinades are used mostly for fish, poultry, or meat, but you can marinate anything, including tofu or vegetables. The result? A mouth-watering meal.
- Brines are solutions of salt, water, and spices that infuse your food with out-of-this-world flavor while tenderizing it and keeping it moist, resulting in a juicier final dish. Brines are usually used for any meat that is not too fatty, such as chicken, turkey, or pork chops. You can brine your food for fifteen minutes to as long as

twenty-four hours. You can also do a "dry brine" by salting meat and letting it soak in the refrigerator. A dry brine works well for many cuts of beef, including steaks.

Beyond Basic Vinaigrette

Once you master this vinaigrette recipe, you can experiment with different vinegars, such as white wine vinegar or rice vinegar, as well as different oils, such as sesame oil or avocado oil, squeezes of lime or lemon, and minced fresh herbs.

> ¼ teaspoon diced garlic (or one small garlic clove, crushed
> and diced)
> 2 tablespoons red wine vinegar
> 2 teaspoons Dijon mustard
> ½ cup olive oil
> Kosher salt and freshly ground black pepper

Whisk the garlic, vinegar, and mustard in a small bowl. Gradually whisk in the oil until emulsified; season with salt and pepper. Transfer to a jar; cover and chill for up to two days.

MAKE YOUR EGGS "EGG-STRA" SPECIAL

There's more to eggs than scrambled eggs! And eggs aren't just for breakfast; you can eat them for lunch, as a snack, or even for dinner.

Fried Eggs

Put a nonstick skillet on medium heat and swirl in a little butter or olive oil. Crack an egg into an individual bowl and slide the egg into the pan.

When the edges turn white, cover the skillet and lower the heat. Wait four minutes (or a couple minutes longer if you want a harder yolk) and season with salt and pepper to taste.

Tip: *Try a fried egg on top of steamed asparagus,*
a salad, or cauliflower rice.

Hard-Boiled Eggs

Place eggs in a large pot and cover with water. Bring the water to a boil over medium heat, then turn off the heat and cover with a lid. If you want soft-boiled eggs, set your kitchen timer for seven minutes. If you want hard-boiled eggs, set your kitchen timer for eleven minutes. Fill a large bowl with ice water, and when the kitchen timer goes off, transfer the eggs to the ice water to stop the cooking process. Remove the eggs after a minute or two.

Tip: *Hard-boiled eggs make "egg-celent" grab-and-go snacks,*
or you can chop them up and add them to a salad or make
deviled eggs or egg salad.

Omelet

In a small bowl, whisk two eggs and season with salt and pepper. In a medium nonstick skillet, melt 2 tablespoons of butter over medium heat. Pour in the eggs and tilt the pan so the eggs cover the entire pan. As the eggs start to set, use a rubber spatula to drag the cooked edges to the center of the pan, and tilt the pan to let the uncooked egg slide to the edge of the pan. Once the bottom is almost set, sprinkle your choice of cheese and chopped fresh herbs (such as chives) on one half of the omelet. Fold one side over the other and slide onto a plate.

....
Tip: Omelets are great for lunch or dinner and make excellent use of whatever chopped veggies (tomatoes, mushrooms, bell pepper, or others) or diced cooked meat (ham, steak, or chicken) you happen to have on hand.
....

Poached Eggs

Fill a saucepan about two-thirds full of water and bring to a boil. Turn the heat down until the water is at a brisk simmer. Crack an egg into a small cup. You can add 1 tablespoon of mild-tasting vinegar to the water (this is optional). Slowly ease the egg into the water. Cook for about 4 minutes and use a slotted spoon to remove the egg from the water. Season to taste with salt and pepper.

....
Tip: Add a poached egg to a salad or cauliflower rice bowl, or use as a topper for asparagus or a burger or on a slice of avocado toast.
....

Yay for Eggs!

Maybe one of the most heavily debated topics in nutrition, eggs have gone from public health enemy number one to being recognized as an important dietary component. What made eggs such a contentious food in the nutrition world was their cholesterol content and unfounded fears that dietary cholesterol negatively impacts heart health. The truth is, you actually need cholesterol to survive, and for the majority of the population, dietary cholesterol does not affect blood cholesterol levels. If you don't have enough cholesterol in your diet, your liver will simply make more, so limiting your dietary cholesterol doesn't do much for your cholesterol levels. Cholesterol is a crucial component of cell membranes, helping transmit signals from one cell to another, and is essential for normal cellular function. It is also used by your body for hormone production and to fight infection. Cholesterol is the precursor to the production of hormones such as testosterone, estrogen, progesterone, and cortisol.

While the nutrition community oscillates back and forth on how many eggs a day are okay to consume, I view eggs, especially their yolks, as nature's multivitamin, as they contain numerous crucial nutrients such as high-quality protein, brain-building choline, lutein, B vitamins, and the fat-soluble vitamins A and E. Eggs actually pair well with a low-carb approach. In fact, one study found that whole eggs combined with a low-carb diet reduced inflammation more than egg whites combined with a low-carb diet.

ESSENTIAL COOKING TECHNIQUES FOR THE HOME COOK

Searing

Bring a steak to room temperature, so it will cook evenly. Set a heavy skillet (cast iron is ideal) over high heat for 2 to 3 minutes. Sprinkle salt into the skillet, then add the steak. Sear for 3 to 4 minutes on each side, until browned on the outside and medium rare on the inside. Remove from heat and let the meat rest on a plate for at least 5 minutes before eating.

Tip: It usually takes about thirty minutes to bring a steak to room temperature.

Sautéing

This method of cooking falls somewhere between stir-frying and searing. Add your choice of butter or oil to a skillet on medium-high heat. Add your choice of food, from scallops or poultry to vegetables or meat; stir or toss until the food is browned slightly and cooked through.

Stir-frying

This method is used for many Asian dishes. To start, make sure every ingredient is fully prepped and cut into bite-size pieces, so they will cook evenly. Add some oil to a large skillet or wok and turn the heat to high. Add the ingredients in order of the ones that take the longest to cook, finishing with the shortest-cooking ingredients so everything is done at the same time. Keep moving the food while you cook it, either with a utensil or by shaking the skillet.

Braising

Braising is good for whole cuts of meat or pieces of chicken that benefit from long, slow cooking to become tender. The food is often, though not necessarily, browned first, and then it is cooked in a low oven or over low heat with a moderate amount of liquid (not enough to cover the food). Use a lid to cover the pot so that liquid condenses on the underside of the lid and keeps the food moist while it cooks. Braising liquids range from broth to wine to tomatoes. Vegetables such as carrots, onions, and other seasonings are often added.

Stewing

Stewing is similar to braising but uses food that has been cut into smaller pieces. The food is usually browned first over higher heat, then returned to the pot with other ingredients, such as vegetables, and liquid to cover. The pot is then partially covered, and the cooking is finished over low heat. Like braising, stewing is an excellent method of tenderizing tougher cuts of meats or poultry or even certain kinds of seafood, such as conch or squid. A slow cooker is the perfect tool for stewing.

Steaming

Steaming is a moist cooking method that works great for chicken, vegetables, and fish. The food is cooked above liquid instead of being submerged, which helps preserve the nutrients in the food. Water is often used, though broth, wine, and beer can also be used. If you don't have a steamer or a steamer basket, you can put a metal colander in a large pot. Make sure the liquid level is about one or two inches below the food; you can add more liquid as it evaporates.

Baking

Baking simply means cooking food in the oven—usually uncovered— using indirect dry heat. Breads, cookies, or muffins, as well as savory food such as lasagna, chicken, or egg dishes are usually baked. The foods cook from the outside in, and the oven temperature varies from recipe to recipe, though once the heat gets to 400°F or above the term *roasting* is often used.

Roasting

Roasting is an easy "hands-off" cooking technique that is similar to baking but uses higher heat and shorter cooking times. You'll use a relatively shallow baking pan so the heat circulates evenly. Vegetables, chicken, and meat are all great for roasting.

Broiling

Broiling involves cooking foods under a broiler, usually on the top rack of your oven, closest to the heat source. The closer the rack is to the heat, the faster it will brown and cook. Fish, seafood, chicken breasts, burgers, and kebabs are good for broiling.

A CUT ABOVE: YOUR ULTIMATE GUIDE TO STEAK

Red meat is rich in vitamins B_{12}, B_3, and B_6, plus selenium, protein, and monounsaturated fat. Grass-fed beef, although pricier, has more omega-3 polyunsaturated fats than grain-fed beef. It's true that red meat has gotten a bad rap in the past due to its supposed link to an increase in heart disease, stroke, and diabetes, but a robust review of the evidence concluded that red meat consumption has little or no effect on major cardiovascular, metabolic, or cancer mortality or incidence.

It was also thought that the saturated fats in red meat increase your LDL ("bad") cholesterol level, which leads to cardiovascular disease, among other illnesses. Though consuming saturated fats may increase your LDL cholesterol level, when your entire diet is taken into consideration, there is no link between saturated fat and cardiovascular disease. And when you consume saturated fat on Atkins 100, where your body is burning primarily fat for fuel, published research has shown that the level of saturated fat in the blood does not increase.

Making the Grade

How do you pick the right cut of meat? First, look for marbling, which is visible streaks of fat that run through the steak and add moisture and flavor. In terms of tenderness, how much fat the cut has, the location of the cut (the loin and rib are the most tender because they are the least used muscles), and the age of the animal at slaughter all come into consideration.

Look for a steak that is 1½ to 2 inches thick. Thin steaks tend to overcook. You want a steak that's thick enough to have a nice sear on the outside while staying tender and juicy on the inside.

The US Department of Agriculture (USDA) divides beef into three grades:

- **Prime:** This includes only 2 percent of all meat and is the most expensive. It is usually sold to restaurants, specialty butchers, and high-end grocery stores, and it is harder to find. It has the most marbling and is great for grilling, as well as roasting or broiling.
- **Choice:** This is probably the best overall for price, tenderness, and marbling.
- **Select:** This is still a high-quality cut of red meat, but it is very lean, which means it has less marbling. It is tender but has less flavor and juiciness than Prime or Choice.

Grass-fed beef typically has less marbling and is leaner than grain-fed beef.

When it comes to grilling, some cuts of beef to look for are:

- **Rib-eye:** This is often considered the most flavorful cut and is very juicy, although it is usually less tender.
- **Filet mignon:** This is the most tender, but it does not have as much flavor as rib-eye.
- **Strip steak:** This is a favorite of steak houses. It is tender and flavorful, with good marbling.
- **Porterhouse/T-bone:** This is extremely tender and great for grilling.
- **Sirloin:** This is usually less tender but very flavorful.

YOUR LOW-CARB GRILLING GUIDE

Grilling is another excellent cooking technique for delicious and easy low-carb meals. Pair your main dish with sides such as grilled asparagus, mushrooms, and zucchini or spinach salad. You can also experiment with different marinades, brines, and spice rubs.

Burgers

Heat a gas grill to high. Brush burgers with olive oil and grill until brown and slightly charred on one side, usually about 3 minutes for beef and 5 minutes for turkey. Flip the burgers and cook beef burgers until brown and slightly charred on the second side, usually 4 minutes for medium rare, until desired degree of doneness. Cook turkey burgers until thoroughly cooked through, about 5 minutes on the second side.

Fish

You can grill fish such as tuna, salmon, halibut, and swordfish directly on the grill, while more delicate fish such as tilapia, sole, and flounder do better in a foil packet or grill basket. Place the fish on a large plate and wrap in paper towels to absorb excess moisture while you are getting the grill ready. Preheat the grill to high and scrape the grill grate clean with a brush. Brush the fish with olive oil and season with kosher salt and freshly ground black pepper or spices of your choice. Place the fish skin side down on the grill. Lower the heat to medium, cover the grill, and let the fish cook. Don't move the fish until the skin looks crisp. You can check by gently lifting the fish with a thin spatula after a few minutes. If it doesn't lift off the grill easily, let it cook a little longer and check again. When the skin is seared and crispy, gently flip the fish using a fork or spatula. Cover and cook until the fish is firm to the touch, flakes easily with a fork, and appears opaque all the way through.

Fresh Produce

Most of your favorite fresh produce can be grilled at medium heat, uncovered, for 2 to 5 minutes. Season with olive oil, kosher salt, and freshly ground pepper before throwing onto the grill. Cut bell peppers into 2-inch strips; cut eggplant, summer squash, and zucchini into ½-inch-thick slices. Mushrooms and cherry tomatoes can also be cooked in a foil pouch for up to 10 minutes.

Pork

Choose pork chops that are about 1½ inches thick. Marinate, brine, or season the chops with spices and/or herbs. When they are ready to grill, pat them dry with paper towels and brush with olive oil and season with kosher salt and freshly ground black pepper. Heat one side of a gas grill at high heat. Keep the other side at low or no heat. Place the chops on the high-heat side of the grill and cook until both sides are brown. Then move them to the low-heat side of the grill to finish cooking. When the internal temperature is 135°F, remove from the grill and let stand for 10 minutes, checking that the internal temperature is at least 145°F.

Poultry

- **Boneless chicken breasts:** Brush with olive oil and season with kosher salt and freshly ground black pepper, or use your choice of marinade, brine, or rub. Grill on a gas grill over medium high for 6 to 8 minutes on each side with the lid closed. Once the internal temperature reaches 165°F, transfer the breasts to a plate and let stand for 5 minutes.
- **Bone-in chicken:** Some people prefer bone-in chicken because it's more flavorful. A budget-friendly option is to start with a whole cut-up chicken on the bone, with skin. Once you have seasoned

the chicken (with marinade, brine, or spices), bring it to room temperature. Heat one side of a gas grill at high heat. Keep the other side at low or no heat. Pat the chicken dry and place bone side down on the low-heat section. Close the grill and let cook for about 20 minutes. Open the grill, turn the pieces over, and cook for about another 15 minutes, until the skin is crispy and the internal temperature is 150 to 155°F. Move the chicken to the high-heat part of the grill to crisp up the skin, and remove it when it reaches an internal temperature of 160°F. Let it rest for 5 to 10 minutes before eating.

Steak

Choose a cut of steak that is at least 1½ inches thick, with marbling in the meat. The fat adds a pop of flavor and makes the steak tender and juicy. The steak should be at or close to room temperature when you cook it so that it will cook evenly. Trim any excess fat off the steak and brush all over with olive oil. Season with kosher salt and pepper.

Preheat the grill to high. Place the steaks on the grill and cook until golden brown and slightly charred, usually about 4 to 5 minutes. Turn the steaks over and continue to grill 3 to 5 minutes for medium rare (an internal temperature of 135°F), 5 to 7 minutes for medium (140°F), or 8 to 10 minutes for medium well done (150°F).

Move the steaks to a cutting board or platter, tent loosely with foil, and let rest for 5 minutes before slicing. This will let the juices distribute throughout the steak. Keep in mind that the steaks will continue to cook while they rest.

If you choose a leaner or grass-fed cut of meat with less marbling, cook it a lower temperature, which will help ensure that it doesn't overcook and dry out. Remove the steak from the grill 10 degrees before it hits the desired temperature. Use an instant-read or meat thermometer for the most accurate results.

LOW-CARB SWAPS FOR HIGH-CARB SIDE DISHES

Whether your main course is a juicy steak, a hamburger hot off the grill, or tender marinated chicken, you'll want to pair it with a side dish. With Atkins 100, no side dish is off limits. Here, you can see how portion sizes and Net Carbs measure up for traditional sides, plus lower-carb swaps for Atkins 40 and Atkins 20.

Side Dish	Serving Size and Net Carbs for Atkins 100	Lower-Carb Swap for Atkins 40	Lower-Carb Swap for Atkins 20
Mashed potatoes	½ cup: 16 grams Net Carbs	1 cup mashed cauliflower: 6 grams Net Carbs	½ cup mashed cauliflower: 3 grams Net Carbs
Potato chips	1 ounce: 15 grams Net Carbs	1 ounce kale chips: 7 grams Net Carbs	1 ounce zucchini crisps: 2 grams Net Carbs
Brown rice	¼ cup: 11 grams Net Carbs	2 tablespoons: 6 grams Net Carbs	1 cup cauliflower rice: 1 gram Net Carb
Beans	¼ cup chickpeas: 11 grams Net Carbs	¼ cup black beans: 6 grams Net Carbs	¼ cup edamame: 2 grams Net Carbs
Corn cut from cob	½ cup: 13 grams Net Carbs	¼ cup: 6 grams Net Carbs	½ cup chopped red bell pepper: 3 grams Net Carbs
Pasta	½ ounce semolina (about ¼ cup cooked): 11 grams Net Carbs	½ ounce chickpea pasta (about ¼ cup cooked): 6 grams Net Carbs	2 cups zucchini "noodles": 5 grams Net Carbs

KITCHEN GADGETS AND TOOLS

I assume you have typical kitchen essentials on hand, such as a reliable set of knives and cooking and serving utensils such as spoons, spatulas, cutting boards, strainers, mixing bowls, and storage containers. But you might want to consider some of these handy tools, as they will help make low-carb cooking even easier:

- **Air fryer:** This popular kitchen appliance cooks by circulating hot air around food, just like a mini convection oven. An air fryer is fabulous for making anything you cook crispy. Skin-on chicken thighs or wings come out crisp without any breading. You can cook small batches of vegetables such as cauliflower, Brussels sprouts, broccoli, zucchini, or sweet potatoes in less time than it takes to preheat your oven, and they taste delicious and have more flavor than when cooked in a microwave or toaster oven.
- **Cast-iron skillet:** Cast iron boasts excellent heat retention, even heat distribution, and nonstick properties (when well seasoned, as explained below), but it does require more care at first than do other pans.

How to Season Your Cast-Iron Skillet

Scrub well with hot, soapy water. Dry thoroughly. Spread a thin layer of vegetable oil over the skillet and place it upside down on a middle rack in an oven preheated to 375°F. (Place a sheet foil on a lower rack to catch any drips.) Bake 1 hour; let cool in the oven. Your skillet is seasoned and good to go!

- **Dehydrator:** This machine uses low temperatures and a fan to dry food. You can dehydrate vegetables such as kale to make kale chips or meat to make jerky.

- **Immersion blender:** This handheld tool lets you blend ingredients or puree food in the container you are preparing it in. You can puree soups or use it to make whipped cream, mayonnaise, vinaigrettes, or smoothies.
- **Instant Pot:** This is a programmable multifunctional cooker. It works as a pressure cooker, slow cooker, rice cooker, and even yogurt maker. If you need a fast, easy dinner to throw together at the last minute or a slow cooker to have dinner waiting when you get home, an Instant Pot adjusts no matter what kind of day it is or how much time you have to spend on a meal.
- **Mini food processor:** This gadget lets you dice, chop, and puree your ingredients in minutes.
- **Muffin tins and ramekins:** Both can be a tremendous help when it comes to controlling the size of the portions you serve. Muffin tins in both the 12-muffin size and the minimuffin size are useful when baking with great-tasting alternatives to wheat flour such as flaxseed meal (high in both protein and fiber) or soy flour. Ramekins are wonderful for baked custards, eggs, minicasseroles, and similar dishes. Be sure to get ramekins that can go straight from the freezer to the oven, so you can prepare ahead and freeze for later use.
- **Salad spinner:** This is used to wash and remove excess water from salad greens.
- **Slow cooker:** Prep the ingredients and throw them into your slow cooker in the morning, set the timer, and your meal is ready when you are. It's perfect for soups, stews, casseroles, curries, and roasts.
- **Spiralizer:** You can buy already spiralized "zoodles" in grocery stores, but if you prefer DIY spiralizing at home, a spiralizer is a helpful tool.

NO TIME TO COOK?

You have options! Skip the drive-through and do a drive-by of your grocery store's salad bar and deli section, plus don't forget about the wonderfully versatile rotisserie chicken, which make it easy to throw together no-cook weeknight meals that are both flavorful and satisfying.

FROM THE DELI

- Chicken, tuna, egg, or shrimp salad
- Grilled, roasted, or broiled chicken
- Grilled, roasted, or smoked turkey
- Ham, pastrami, corned beef, salami, brisket
- Rotisserie chicken (of course)
- Sauerkraut, pickles, pickled green beans, pickled mushrooms, cucumber salad, coleslaw

....
Tip: *Be sure to ask questions, read labels, and avoid meats cured with nitrates or made with bread crumbs and other fillers, starchy sauces, and salads with added sugar.*
....

FROM THE SALAD BAR

- Bean salad
- Berries, melon balls, and other fruit
- Grilled, braised, or steamed broccoli, asparagus, cauliflower, and green beans
- Grilled, roasted, or baked turkey, salmon, tuna, and chicken; grilled or steamed shrimp
- Hard-boiled eggs and deviled eggs
- Nuts, seeds, crumbled bacon, grated cheese, and feta or blue cheese crumbles
- Olives, hummus, and baba ghanoush
- Salad greens, tomatoes, avocado, and other salad veggies
- Vinaigrette, blue cheese, or ranch dressing

Tip: Watch out for meats and fish with starchy sauces, croutons, crunchy noodles, and pasta salads, which will boost your carb intake higher than you'd like.

LOW-CARB MEALS FOR BUSY NIGHTS

The easiest way to ensure that you eat the food that's in your fridge is to prep it as soon as you get home. On grocery-shopping day, leave yourself time to wash and chop all your veggies, grill a batch of chicken breasts or thighs, and cook ground beef and turkey for the week ahead. This will make Atkins 100 weeknight eating a no-brainer. Whether you've already stocked your kitchen or you're relying on some quick choices you grabbed from the deli, here are some busy-night meal ideas.

- Top a premade bagged salad with deli turkey, ham, or rotisserie chicken.
- Pick up some rotisserie chicken and a cucumber and tomato salad from the deli.
- **Burger bar:** Grill up some burgers and provide all the fixings. Skip the bun for a lower-carb option.
- **Taco bar:** Reheat ground beef or turkey or shred that rotisserie chicken and throw in avocado, salsa, shredded cheese, and more. Turn your taco into a taco salad for a lower-carb option.
- **Chili bar:** Plan ahead and put your chili makings into your slow cooker or Instant Pot in the morning. Serve with all the fixings, such as avocado, shredded cheese, diced jalapeños for some heat, sour cream, wedges of lime, and chopped cilantro.
- **Salad bar:** Easy-peasy! Pick up salad fixings from your deli (or pull some from your fridge) and let everyone make their own.
- **A family-friendly snack board:** Grab a board or a platter, and you can make dinner time a finger food affair by serving an array of

fun and filling finger foods: cherry tomatoes, sliced cucumber and bell peppers, baby carrots, celery, steamed bite-size pieces of broccoli, green beans, or sugar snap peas, plus slices of deli ham, turkey, and salami and slices or cubes of Swiss, Havarti, Gouda, or cheddar cheese. Use ramekins for hummus, ranch dressing, olives, and nuts. The kids might want crackers and cheese; go for high-fiber crackers, which are lower in carbs.

• **Breakfast for dinner:** See page 112 for egg options. Take whatever veggies and meat you have on hand and toss them into an omelet or top with a poached or fried egg, while sizzling up a little bacon.

Next up? Even if you're killing it in the kitchen, eating out is almost inevitable. With Atkins 100, there are endless low-carb options available to you, whether you're ordering in, enjoying a sit-down meal or flying by the fast-food drive-through. Head to the next chapter to find out how!

CHAPTER 6

LOW-CARB EATING OUT HACKS

If you can't stand the heat, get out of the kitchen.
—President Harry S. Truman

COOKING AT HOME is optimal because you're in control of both the ingredients and the portions. But who doesn't love the treat of having a night out with someone else doing the cooking and dishes? In fact, in 2019, almost 57 percent of Americans ate out or did takeout or delivery at least two to three times a week. Over the years, I've developed some excellent hacks that help me stick with my low-carb lifestyle while enjoying meals everywhere from sit-down restaurants to fast-food and fast-casual restaurants. I even have some hacks up my sleeve for making low-carb choices on the go.

EATING OUT (OR ORDERING IN) BEGINS WITH PLANNING

Though this is a chance to give yourself a break from meal planning, meal prep, and cooking, it's still essential to have a plan no matter how you choose to dine:

- **Review the menu beforehand.** Before I head to a restaurant or order takeout or a delivery, I always pull up the menu online to check my choices. If I'm eating out, I decide what to order before I arrive at the restaurant because that way I'm usually much less swayed by the specials of the day or what everyone else is ordering.
- **Have a snack before you go.** Eating a light snack before you go out to eat or order in can help prevent you from overeating. Choose something that's healthy and filling but won't ruin your appetite, such as veggies and guacamole or a few turkey or ham roll-ups.
- **Drink a couple glasses of water beforehand, too.** This will help fill you up and curb your appetite.

Low-Carb Science Bite

The science of appetite regulation could have its own book! One well-researched tip is to drink water before your meal to help curb your appetite. It's thought that water consumption helps fill you up, and the distension of your stomach sends signals to your brain that you're full. The data suggest that drinking 16 ounces of water about thirty minutes before a meal can help with weight loss. In fact, when this was put into practice in a randomized controlled trial, those in the group who were told to consume water before their meal lost about twice as much weight as those in the control group.

- **Speak your mind.** Don't be afraid to let your server know (politely, of course) if you'd like to make any changes to your order, such as dressing on the side or grilled chicken instead of fried.
- **Watch out for "health" claims on menus.** There are no standards for the terms "low carb" or "healthy."

- **Request sauce and gravy on the side.** You never know how much sugar or starches are in a sauce, and gravy is almost always thickened with flour or cornstarch.
- **Get to know cooking terms.** If chicken or fish is described as crispy on a menu, that usually means it's fried, breaded, or battered. Look for entrees with words such as roasted, grilled, pan-fried, sautéed, or poached.
- **Pare down your portions.** Restaurant portions are notoriously large. Take control of the situation by sharing a dish or saving your leftovers for another meal. Turning one meal into two also makes eating out easier on your wallet!
- **Pass on the bread or chips.** Many restaurants provide complimentary bread or baskets of tortilla chips to start off the meal. Of course, no food is forbidden on Atkins 100, but mindlessly munching on a basket of bread or chips can easily put you over your 100 grams of Net Carbs for the day. If it's a challenge to resist more than a few chips or a little bread dipped in olive oil, politely tell the server that you don't need the basket or ask if it would be possible for them to take it away earlier than usual. If salsa, hummus, or guacamole come with bread or chips, ask if you can substitute sliced veggies instead.
- **Soup's on!** I love soup because it's a great appetite squelcher. Miso soup, cream soup, and clear broth with meat or vegetables are all satisfying and delicious ways to satiate your appetite before the main dish arrives. You can also pair your soup with a salad for a complete meal. (Some cream soups are thickened with flour, so double check with your server first before ordering.)
- **Be smart about sides.** Instead of fries, how about a side salad? Or double up on your vegetables or brown rice or another whole grain.
- **Decide whether to have dessert *before* you order dinner.** If you're not going to have dessert, make sure your entrée is satisfying and

filling enough so you aren't tempted by a sweet treat, especially if your companions are indulging. If you plan to order dessert, skip the bread or pasta and/or stick with berries with whipped cream or melon.

- **Give yourself a break.** Don't torture yourself if you overdo it on the breadbasket or you didn't realize that your entrée would be breaded and fried. The wonderful thing about Atkins 100 is that no food is off limits, and this is just one meal.

Low-Carb Convos with Your Fellow Diners

Compared to years past, low-carb living is top of mind for many people, which makes it a lot easier to make lower-carb choices while you're eating out. Your fellow diners will probably be quite support-ive, or they may be following their own version of a low-carb diet and be curious about Atkins 100. Though the last thing you want to do is make the meal all about you and your eating habits, you can reframe the conversation in a positive way if it does come up.

LOW-CARB HACKS FOR EVERY CUISINE

If you love eating out or ordering in, with Atkins 100, no matter what cuisine you crave, you have choices. Here are some suggestions for eight popular cuisines:

Chinese

Rice is a staple of all Chinese cuisines, and although there are excep-tions, most Chinese dishes use meat as an addition rather than the main ingredient. In many dishes, minimally cooked fresh vegetables form the bulk of the preparation, with various sauces. A huge country with great geographical diversity, China is blessed with multiple regional cuisines, several of which have taken root in the United States. All of them offer low-carb options for you to enjoy.

Order This	Instead of This
Egg drop soup	Egg rolls
Sizzling shrimp platter	Shrimp fried rice
Steamed tofu with vegetables and sesame, garlic, or black bean sauce	Any chow fun (wide noodle) dish
Stir-fried pork with garlic sauce	Sweet-and-sour pork
Beef with Chinese mushrooms	Beef lo mein
Steamed whole fish	Shrimp with black bean sauce
Chicken with broccoli	Kung pao chicken, sesame chicken, or sweet-and-sour chicken (which is usually deep fried)
Sautéed spinach with garlic	Moo shu vegetables with pancakes

Tip: Many Chinese sauces are prepared with sugar or cornstarch; stick to dishes that are stir-fried, steamed, or broiled.

∙∙∙∙∙∙∙∙∙∙∙∙∙∙∙∙∙∙∙∙∙∙∙∙∙∙∙∙∙∙∙

Tip: If you nix the pancakes or stick to just one, moo shu vegetables or moo shu pork is perfectly acceptable on Atkins 100.

∙∙∙∙∙∙∙∙∙∙∙∙∙∙∙∙∙∙∙∙∙∙∙∙∙∙∙∙∙∙∙

Tip: Instead of white rice, ask for a small serving of brown rice.

∙∙∙∙∙∙∙∙∙∙∙∙∙∙∙∙∙∙∙∙∙∙∙∙∙∙∙∙∙∙∙

French

French cuisine is actually a collection of regional specialties determined by climate, geology, and proximity to the sea. You'll find fish, herbs, and olives in Provence; butter and apples in Normandy; wine for simmering stews in Burgundy and Bordeaux; sausages and beer in Alsace. There's a huge variety of cheese everywhere, and you'll be happy to know that many French sauces are perfectly acceptable because they're based on butter or olive oil and thickened with egg yolks rather than flour. For example, asparagus with hollandaise sauce is naturally low in carbs and remarkably delicious.

Order This	Instead of This
Frisée salad with lardons (thin strips of bacon) and poached egg	Alsatian tart (a bacon, onion, and egg pie)
Coquilles St. Jacques (scallops in cream sauce with cheese)	Langoustine en croûte (lobster in puff pastry)
Moules marinières (mussels in white wine and herbs) or bouillabaisse (fish stew)	Vichyssoise (cream of potato and leek soup)

Coq au vin (chicken in wine sauce)	Caneton à l'orange or aux cerises (duck with oranges or cherries)
Entrecôte or tournedos Bordelaise (steak in reduced shallot and red wine sauce)	Croque monsieur (egg-dipped fried ham-and-egg sandwich)
Veal Marengo (veal stew with tomatoes and mushrooms)	Veal Prince Orloff (veal roast stuffed with rice, onions, and mushrooms)
Haricots verts au beurre (buttered young green beans)	Pommes Anna (upside-down potato cake)
Assorted cheese plate	Crêpes Suzette (crêpes with orange butter and orange liquor, served flambéed)

Tip: It's okay to order dishes containing butter and cream, but simpler dishes such as fish Provençal with tomatoes and herbs or steak au poivre are smarter choices.

Tip: Beware of pommes frites, or French fries. They are almost irresistible and often accompany steak dishes. Make sure to request a side salad or vegetable instead.

Indian

Indian cuisines are complex and contain multiple ingredients. In general, healthy options include kebabs, tandoori, and meat curry, which derive their flavor from herbs and spices. Try raita, which is yogurt mixed with minced cucumbers, to ease the heat of some of the more powerful curries.

Order This	Instead of This
Shahi paneer or saag paneer (homemade cheese in creamy tomato sauce or cooked spinach, cheese, and spices)	Vegetable samosas (deep-fried pastries)
Roasted eggplant with onions and spices	Pakora (fritter)
Chicken shorba soup (made with garlic, ginger, cinnamon, and other spices)	Lentil or mulligatawny soup
Korma (meat in cream sauce)	Biryani (rice dish)
Tandoori chicken or shrimp	Chicken or shrimp vindaloo
Lamb or chicken curry	Dal (lentil or bean dish)

Tip: When in doubt, ask what's in a dish. Many curries, as well as vindaloos, contain potatoes.

....

Tip: *Indian cuisine features a variety of delicious breads, such as naan, chapati, poori, and paratha. If you can't stick to one piece, ask for spiced cooked vegetables or a cooked cheese dish such as shahi paneer.*

....

Tip: *You can't go wrong with lamb, chicken, or shrimp kebabs or lamb, chicken, or shrimp saag. Saag consists of greens such as spinach or mustard greens that are simmered with onion, garlic, spices, and heavy cream or butter.*

....

Italian

Italy has a rich and varied culinary heritage that goes far beyond the southern Italian food we're generally used to. Northern Italian food is reminiscent of French cuisine without the pretensions. It features rich butter and cream sauces, highly developed flavors, and carefully prepared fresh ingredients. Tuscan foods are prepared to emphasize the essential flavors of individual ingredients. The signature element in Florentine dishes is spinach, and from the French border to Venice, you're unlikely to find pasta on the menu at all. Instead, rice dishes called risotti or cornmeal dishes called polenta are the regional starches.

Order This	Instead of This
Insalata di frutti di mare (seafood salad)	Deep-fried calamari
Mixed grilled vegetables or sautéed portobello mushrooms	Deep-fried mozzarella sticks

Antipasto (assorted meats and cheeses); marinated peppers and mushrooms	Baked stuffed clams
Escarole soup or stracciatella (an Italian egg drop soup with spinach, egg, and Parmesan)	Fettucine Alfredo
Roasted red snapper or salmon; grilled calamari or shrimp scampi	Linguine with clam sauce
Grilled chicken paillard (boneless chicken breast, pounded thin) or pork loin	Risotto
Veal or chicken piccata or scallopini with lemon and capers	Veal, chicken, or eggplant Parmesan

Tip: Order a dish of olives instead of the breadbasket.

Tip: Start your meal with a bowl of soup, such as a clear broth or stracciatella.

Japanese

Japan, an island nation, has many seafood dishes prepared in a variety of ways. But a number of other protein sources have also found their way into Japanese cuisine, as well as a vast variety of fresh vegetables and flavor profiles that include shoyu soy sauce, which is milder and sweeter than Chinese soy sauce, nutty flavors from sesame seeds and sesame oil, plus seaweed, fish flakes, and pickled ginger.

Order This	Instead of This
Pickled vegetables and/or miso soup	Edamame
Steamed vegetables or grilled Japanese eggplant	Gyoza (fried dumplings)
Shabu-shabu (thin slices of beef and vegetables that you cook at the table in a broth)	Sukiyaki (beef, vegetables, tofu, and noodles simmered in a sweet sauce)
Broiled fish	Shrimp tempura
Grilled squid	Seafood noodle dishes
Negimaki (scallions or asparagus tips wrapped in paper-thin slices of beef dipped in soy sauce)	Beef teriyaki
Sashimi (artfully sliced raw fish)	Sushi (sliced raw fish arranged on rice)

Mexican

There's much more to Mexican cuisine than tortillas, beans, and rice. The primary flavor components of Mexican food are garlic, chiles, cilantro, and cumin. Depending on the region of Mexico, you'll find everything from seafood-focused dishes to dishes with a French influence, as well as an emphasis on fresh vegetables.

Order This	Instead of This
Grilled chicken wings with ranch dressing	Chiles rellenos
Sopa de albóndigas (meatball and vegetable soup)	Quesadilla
Jicama salad	Nachos
Grilled pescado special (fresh fish of the day) with grilled vegetables and chilies or mixed seafood (mariscos)	Taco platter
Pollo asado (grilled marinated chicken) with pico de gallo	Chicken chimichanga
Camarones al ajillo (shrimp in garlic sauce)	Shrimp enchilada
Grilled skirt steak with onion and chilies	Beef burrito
Turkey or chicken mole	Chicken tostada, enchilada, or tamales

Tip: Skip the traditional bowl of tortilla chips and salsa and order guacamole with jicama or cucumber slices for dipping.

Tip: Nix the premixed margarita in favor of a lower-carb version made with tequila, lime juice, and triple sec.

Middle Eastern

Popular dishes in Middle Eastern restaurants include rice, chickpeas, and lentils. Eggplant also gets star treatment. But there are also a number of meat dishes, especially lamb-based ones, and baba ghanoush, roasted eggplant that's mashed and mixed with garlic and tahini, a paste made from sesame seeds. Traditionally, it is eaten with flatbread, but you can substitute celery sticks, green pepper chunks, or even onion chunks.

Order This	Instead of This
Loubieh bi zeit (green beans braised in olive oil with tomatoes) or baba ghanoush	Tabbouleh (bulgur salad)
Eggplant with garlic, tomatoes, and peppers	Fattoush (ground lamb and bulgur patties)
Shish kebab (grilled spiced cubed lamb on skewers)	Kibbe (ground lamb and bulgur patties)
Kofta balls of ground lamb and onions, skewered and grilled	Falafel (chickpea patties)

| Shish taouk (skewered pieces of marinated chicken grilled over charcoal) | B'steeya (Moroccan chicken pie with almonds) |

. . . .

Tip: *Start your meal with a glass of Middle Eastern mint tea.*
It will fill you up and help digestion.

. . . .

Tip: *If you order the thickened labneh yogurt flavored*
with mint or hummus as an appetizer, ask for raw
vegetables to dip instead of pita bread.

. . . .

Thai

Thai food is a blend of Chinese and Indian culinary traditions, with the brightness of tropical colors and flavors as well as unique seasonings and condiments. For a small country, Thailand has a lengthy coastline, so seafood is plentiful, but as in most other countries in that part of the world, meat is scarce and costly, so chefs rely heavily on rice and noodles. The flavors and combinations that make Thai food distinctive— including coconut milk, lemongrass, tamarind, cilantro, turmeric, cumin, chilies, lime juice, and kaffir lime leaves—can be found in plenty of other dishes that aren't based on noodles or rice.

Order This	Instead of This
Tom yum koong (shrimp and mushrooms simmered in hot-and-sour broth with coriander, lime leaves, and lemongrass) or gai tom kha (a soup made with chicken slices simmered in coconut milk)	Dumplings or spring rolls

Sautéed shrimp or beef with basil, onions, and chilies	Pad thai
Sautéed scallops and shrimp (or beef or pork) with mushrooms, zucchini, and chili paste	Any curry dish
Sautéed beef, chicken, or pork with shrimp paste and green beans	Sautéed beef, chicken, or pork with ginger, black bean sauce, and green onion
Sautéed mixed vegetables	Thai fried rice with vegetables
Steamed mussels with herbs and garlic sauce	Deep-fried whole fish with sweet-and-sour sauce

....

Tip: Avoid black bean thread noodles and other noodles.

....

Tip: Anything listed as pad *on the menu is usually stir-fried with noodles or rice; look for options with a protein base.*

....

Tip: Instead of white rice, order a small serving of brown rice, if available.

....

Curious About Cocktails on Atkins 100?

When you're eating out, it's tempting to enjoy a cocktail or two with your meal, and you certainly can on Atkins 100. Just be sure to count the grams of Net Carbs in the drink as part of your day's total intake. Here are my tips for making the best carb-conscious cocktail choices:

- **Get spirited.** *Certain spirits—such as Scotch, rye, vodka, and gin—are naturally low in carbs. Just be sure to avoid mixing them with juice, tonic water, or nondiet soda. Go for seltzer, diet tonic, or diet soda instead.*
- **Wine also wins.** *If you'd prefer white wine, pinot grigio and sauvignon blanc are your best choices. If you're into red, try pinot noir. A 5-ounce glass of wine contains a little more than 3 grams of Net Carbs. If you're in the mood for a little bubbly, there's good news: champagne or sparkling wine contains anywhere from 1.5 to 2.5 grams of Net Carbs per 5-ounce glass. Choose dry varieties of wine instead of sweet wines, which tend to be higher in carbs. There are new low-carb brands of wine and beer on the market that are worth checking out. As always, don't forget to add these carbs to your total daily count.*
- **Mix it up.** *A mixed drink such as a martini, a "skinny" margarita, vodka and soda with a splash of lime, or gin and (diet) tonic are lower in carbs. Consider any of those options over fruity mixed drinks such as a frozen margarita, a daiquiri, Long Island iced tea, a mojito, or the king of all sugary mixed drinks, a piña colada, which could contain up to 60 grams of sugar!*
- **Water works.** *Alcohol can dehydrate you, and dehydration is also the culprit for hangovers everywhere, so follow each alcoholic beverage with a glass of water or club soda.*
- **A little goes a long way!** *One too many drinks, and suddenly it's not as easy to resist the tempting treats that surround you.*

Your body will also burn alcohol before fat, so if you overdo it, it may slow down weight loss.

- **Make it a mocktail.** *More companies have started to offer zero-alcohol beer (that actually tastes good!) and mocktail mixes, and bars are starting to include mocktails on their menus, if you want to feel as though you're imbibing while keeping your wits about you. A word of caution: you may not miss the booze in your mocktail, but if it's made with fruit juice or simple syrup, it's probably full of sugar. Stick with mocktails that contain sugar-free fruit-flavored sparkling water, blends, and garnishes of low-glycemic fruits such as berries, sweeteners such as stevia or sucralose, and a squeeze of fresh lime or lemon juice.*

LOW-CARB HACKS FOR FAST-FOOD RESTAURANTS

Fast food is a fact of life, but most items tend to be high in calories and carbs and low in nutrients. Though you have more control over the quality of food when you prepare it at home, sometimes fast food is your only option, whether you're on the road or need a quick meal. Here are my fast-food hacks, plus my suggestions for what to order at popular fast-food restaurants.

SEVEN HACKS FOR ORDERING FAST FOOD

1. **Skip the bun.** Some establishments let you order a burger wrapped in lettuce leaves, or you can always remove the bun and eat the inside with a fork.
2. **Avoid fried food.** Some chains now offer grilled, broiled, or roasted chicken that's neither battered nor breaded. In a pinch, peel the battered skin off of a piece of fried chicken or fish and eat only the meat. Limit your consumption of French fries, which are high in trans fats; studies show that eating them may trigger cravings for more.

3. **Get dressing on the side.** Sauces and salad dressings may be full of sugar or corn syrup. Check the ingredients, have it on the side, or even bring your own.

4. **Fill up on veggies.** Head to the salad bar or choose a salad from the menu. Top your salad with proteins such as ham or chicken and healthy fats such as sunflower seeds.

5. **Check nutritional info.** Most chains provide complete nutritional data for their foods online.

6. **Skip the value meal.** Though a value meal may seem budget friendly, your healthiest bet is to order à la carte, so you resist the temptation of a meal that includes fries and a sugary soft drink.

7. **Watch your portions.** There's no need to supersize. Share your meal with friends, or portion out half when your food arrives, leaving the other half to take home.

Fast-Food Meals: Eat This, Not That

Here are my suggestions for what to eat and what not to eat when you're contemplating your next trip through the drive-through. Keep in mind that just one of these items (although it seems small) might easily count as an Atkins 100 meal, coming in at close to 25 grams of Net Carbs; a suggested small side could be a snack at 10 to 15 grams of Net Carbs. Be sure to choose wisely and ask yourself if it makes sense to blow a whole meal on four chicken tenders or one taco when you can order a salad with grilled chicken.

Tip: You can use the Atkins Mobile Weight Loss Tracker & Carb Counter app to help formulate your meal plan before going to a fast-food restaurant, or check out the nutritional values for each menu item on the restaurant's website.

Calculating Fast-Food Carbs

Be sure to go online and double-check the nutritional informa-tion for your fast-food choices, as menu items might change. Here's how to plan for Atkins 100, Atkins 40, and Atkins 20:

Atkins 100

• *Main dishes generally contain no more than 18 grams of Net Carbs per serving. Appetizers, soups, sides, snacks, and desserts generally contain no more than 12 grams of Net Carbs per serving*

Atkins 40

• *Main dishes generally contain no more than 12 grams of Net Carbs per serving. Appetizers, soups, sides, snacks, and desserts generally contain no more than 9 grams of Net Carbs per serving.*

Atkins 20

• *Main dishes generally contain no more than 7 grams of Net Carbs per serving. Appetizers, soups, sides, snacks, and desserts generally contain no more than 3 grams of Net Carbs per serving.*

Arby's

Eat this: *Minus the bun*: Roast chicken, roast turkey, roast ham, roast beef, roast beef melts, reuben corned beef, and BLT sandwiches and the contents of all subs; sliders except buffalo chicken and chicken tender; Chopped Farmhouse Salad with Roasted Turkey and Chopped Side Salad with buttermilk ranch dressing

Not that: Chicken tenders; crispy and buffalo chicken salads and sandwiches; most salad dressings and condiments

Burger King

Eat this: *Minus the bun*: All burgers and Whoppers; four-piece and six-piece spicy or regular chicken nuggets; the crispy taco; breakfast burrito, jr.; garden side salad and Ken's ranch dressing

Not that: Crispy chicken; crispy garden salad; chicken tenders; honey mustard and Ken's fat-free ranch dressings

Carl's Jr.

Eat this: Low-Carb Charbroiled Chicken Club; *minus the bun*: Famous Star, Big Carl, Guacamole Bacon Burger, most other burgers/cheeseburgers, and Charbroiled Chicken Club and Charbroiled Chicken Santa Fe Chicken sandwiches; crunchy beef and chicken soft tacos; three-piece and five-piece chicken tenders; the charbroiled chicken salad (lose the croutons); side salad; house and blue cheese salad dressings; house and buffalo wing sauces

Not that: Teriyaki burger; parmesan chicken sandwich; all other fried chicken and fish dishes; Thousand Island and low-fat balsamic salad dressings; BBQ, honey, mustard, and sweet-and-sour sauces

Chick-fil-A

Eat this: *Minus the biscuit*: Breakfast egg, cheese, sausage, and bacon dishes; sausage breakfast burrito (unwrap and discard the tortilla); Hash Brown Scramble Bowl; fruit cup; nuggets and grilled nuggets; chicken strips; grilled chicken and grilled chicken club sandwiches (minus the bread); southwest, cobb, and market salads (with grilled chicken or grilled fillet); blue cheese, Caesar, and buttermilk ranch salad dressings; Buffalo and buttermilk ranch sauces

Not that: All breaded and fried chicken dishes; Chick-fil-A sauce; barbecue, honey mustard, and Polynesian sauces; fat-free honey mustard and other low-fat or no-fat salad dressings

Dairy Queen

Eat this: *Minus the bun*: Grillburgers, hamburgers, cheeseburgers, hot dogs, cheese dogs, grilled chicken and turkey items; side salad; chicken BLT salad (with grilled chicken); BBQ, wild buffalo, and ranch dipping sauces

Not that: All crispy chicken items; blue cheese, sweet-and-sour, and honey mustard dipping sauces; all fat-free salad dressings; sadly, all DQ ice cream is naturally high in carbs and sugar

Hardee's

Eat this: Hardee's Better for You Options menu: Low-carb Thickburger and Charbroiled Chicken Club Sandwich; side salad; three-piece or five-piece chicken tenders

Not that: All other burgers with buns

In-N-Out Burger

Eat this: Any burger "animal style," meaning without the bun

Not that: Burger with the bun; French fries; shakes

KFC

Eat this: Caesar side salad or side salad; grilled chicken; Original Fried Chicken (the Extra Crispy, Spicy Crispy and Nashville Hot options tend to have more carbs); most wing dishes; green beans

Not that: All fried, breaded, or crispy dishes; biscuits; most sides

McDonald's

Eat this: Any breakfast sandwich without the bun or biscuit; any burger without the bun (or go for the regular hamburger or cheeseburger); any grilled chicken sandwich without the bun; grilled chicken salads; side salad

Not that: French fries; McCafe coffee drinks; shakes; McFlurry shakes, sundaes, and cones

Taco Bell

Eat this: Power Menu Bowl (minus the rice and beans); Power Menu Veggie Bowl (minus the rice and beans); Fiesta Taco Salad (don't eat the shell bowl); Mini Skillet Bowl (no potatoes); Fresco Soft Taco Chicken; Fresco Soft Taco Beef; Fresco Soft Taco Steak; Fresco Crispy Taco Beef; Pintos n Cheese; Black Beans; Cheesy Roll Up; Meximelt; Spicy Tostada; soft taco; crunchy taco

Not that: Black Bean Quesarito (coming in at a whopping 73 grams of Net Carbs!); most burritos, chalupas, crunchwraps, nachos, and quesadillas

LOW-CARB HACKS FOR FAST-CASUAL RESTAURANTS

A fast-casual restaurant does not offer full table service but typically features higher-quality food than fast-food restaurants do, with fewer frozen or processed ingredients. It is usually more expensive than fast food, but you generally have your pick of healthier options, including low-carb and keto selections. Since your meal is made in front of you, this allows you the chance to customize it as well.

Chipotle

Eat this: Make your own burrito bowl or salad by adding the meat of your choice, piling on fajita vegetables and salad greens, going with a garnish or small portion of beans or rice, and adding flavor with salsas, guacamole, sour cream, and cheese.

Not that: Any of the burritos, tacos, or quesadillas—due to the high-carb, extra-large tortillas that come with them. Also avoid chips, corn salsa, sofritos, and full servings of beans and rice. Be cautious not to add on too many "extras," as their Net Carbs do add up quickly.

....
Tip: *See Appendices A through D for recommended portion sizes and Net Carbs of foods such as beans and rice.*
....

Noodles

Eat this: Anything with zucchini "zoodles," a small salad, a side salad, or a side of any soup.

Not that: Any dishes with noodles, which weigh in big on carbs.

Panera Bread

Eat this: Strawberry Poppyseed Salad with Chicken; Caesar Salad with Chicken; Greek Salad; Southwest Chili Lime Ranch Salad with Chicken; Asian Sesame Salad with Chicken; Seasonal Greens Salad; Green Goddess Cobb Salad with Chicken; Low-Fat Chicken Noodle Soup; or any breakfast sandwich without the bread.

Not that: The rest of the soups, sandwiches, and breads.

Smashburger

Eat this: Burgers and grilled chicken sandwiches without the bun; BBQ Ranch Salad (hold the BBQ sauce); cobb salad; side salad; crispy Brussels sprouts.

Not that: Burgers and sandwiches with the bun; French fries; shakes.

Starbucks

Eat this: The protein and snack boxes; a protein bowl; any breakfast sandwich without a bun or biscuit; sous vide egg bites. Order coffee drinks with sugar-free syrup, heavy cream, or unsweetened nut milk instead of regular milk.

Not that: Any of the pastries, scones, brownies, or cookies. When it comes to coffee and tea drinks, do your research and read the nutrition facts. Though an iced green tea sounds healthy, it has 23 grams of sugar, twice as much as a cappuccino.

WHEN THE TIME IS RIGHT: PARTIES AND POTLUCKS

When you're ready to join family and friends for a delicious meal together, a dinner party at someone's home should be relatively easy to navigate with Atkins 100. If the soirée is buffet style, you can master it by sticking with roast turkey, ham, roast beef, salmon fillet, or other protein dishes, as well as tossed salads and Foundation Vegetables. With Atkins 100, you can also enjoy modest portions of sweet potatoes, carrots, or other starchy veggies—or even some whole grain bread. At sitdown meals, there's no rule against simply not serving yourself a food you want to stay away from. If your hostess insists that you try it, take a small portion, have a tiny taste, and leave it at that.

If you're the host or hostess, you are in control. You can prepare a mix of low-carb dishes and ones a little higher in carbs; just make sure you have a small serving of the higher-carb dishes. Or you can do what I love to do: host a dinner party featuring all low-carb recipes. You may be surprised at how receptive everyone is to the delicious array of food, while realizing they aren't missing out on traditional high-carb entrees and sides. I usually share the recipe for each dish, and the same goes if I'm bringing a low-carb dish to a potluck. It adds a personal touch, and it shows people just how easy it is to eat this way. You can start creating the perfect low-carb gathering, whether it's for brunch, lunch, or dinner plus dessert, with our low-carb recipes starting on page 181.

How to Handle the Holidays

With Atkins 100, you have plenty of options when it comes to celebrating the holidays. To start, eat your three meals of 25 grams of Net Carbs and two snacks of 10 to 15 grams of Net Carbs a day to keep your appetite under control. Let's take a look:

• **Thanksgiving:** *Start by filling your plate with turkey, ham, and vegetable side dishes. Stick with smaller servings (or tastes) of* mashed potatoes, sweet potatoes, and stuffing. Take advantage of any leftover turkey or ham and feast on roll-ups, or add the meat to eggs, salads, or soups.

- **Hanukkah:** You can enjoy brisket, but watch your latke intake. As an alternative to potato latkes, try a latke recipe using shredded zucchini. Once again, take advantage of any brisket leftovers.
- **Christmas:** If you're Italian American, the Feast of the Seven Fishes, on Christmas Eve, is your chance to indulge in heart-healthy fish. This holiday also involves dishes featuring turkey, ham, beef, or lamb. Once again, go with smaller portions of potato dishes or stuffing.
- **St. Patrick's Day:** It's not just the luck of the Irish: the traditional main dish of this holiday, corned beef and cabbage, is low in carbs.
- **Easter:** You can eat ham and all the hard-boiled Easter eggs you would like, while taking advantage of spring vegetables such as asparagus, which you can smother in a rich hollandaise sauce. Turn the leftover hard-boiled eggs into egg salad for a quick lunch or deviled eggs for a yummy low-carb snack.
- **Fourth of July:** Skip the buns on your burgers and brats and enjoy all the fresh vegetables that are in season this time of year, including tomatoes, cucumbers, summer squash, and even corn on the cob in moderation. Indulge in small servings or tastes of high-carb side dishes such as pasta salad.

WHEN YOU'RE ON THE ROAD

If you travel for business, your usual schedule of meals and snacks is bound to change based on where you are and what's available. If you're on vacation, the same applies, with the additional temptation of local cuisine and drinks.

On a Plane or Train

Whether you're flying or taking a train, pack some low-carb snacks (page 249), as well as a refillable water bottle. The airport has its share of fast-food fare (see page 145 to learn what and what not to order). Your in-flight food may be questionable or nonexistent, but many airports also have grab-and-go options at kiosks, where it's possible to pick up salads and snacks such as hard-boiled eggs for your flight.

At a Hotel

Here are some tips for eating in a hotel:

- **The "free" continental breakfast while traveling for business:** Skip the premade waffles and syrup and doughnuts and fill up with scrambled eggs, bacon, sausage, hard-boiled eggs, and low-glycemic berries.
- **A leisurely hotel breakfast on vacation:** Though the freshly made waffles, pancakes, French toast, and pastries will certainly tempt you, choose an omelet or scramble made to order with your choice of fillings, such as diced ham or bacon, sliced mushrooms, tomatoes, chilies, and shredded cheese. Have a side of fresh fruit instead of hash browns or breakfast potatoes.
- **Room service:** Specify what you don't want—no toast with your eggs and no rolls with your dinner order—as well as what you do want. You can politely ask the server to remove the toast, rolls, or side of potatoes on the room service cart if you didn't ask for them. As soon as you're done, put the tray outside the door so you don't wind up grazing on the extras hours later.
- **The minibar:** Resist the impulse to check out its contents. Other than overpriced bottled water, it's a minefield studded with sugary and starchy snacks. If you think you may give in to tempta-

tion, decline the key to the fridge or return it to the reception desk.

Out and About

If you're on vacation, most likely you'll want to partake in the local cuisine, especially if you're in a city with a thriving culinary scene. Here are some tips:

- To enjoy the cuisine without overdoing it, have eggs for breakfast and a salad with protein for lunch. That should leave a bit of a margin to enjoy the local specialty for dinner—in moderation, of course.
- Explore the range of local foods, whether seafood in San Francisco, gumbo in New Orleans, or barbecue in Austin, to name a few. Choose a local specialty that's prepared without breading or starchy sauces. Stick with the eating out tips you've learned so far to set you up for success!

Low-Carb Hacks for Road Trips

Road trips can be fun for the whole family. Whether you go on a cross-country excursion or a long weekend, it's essential to have healthy low-carb snacks readily available so that you avoid the potential dietary pitfalls of convenience stores and fast-food restaurants along your route. Your pit stops don't have to be pitfalls if you follow these tips along the way:

- **Stay hydrated.** *Skip the sugary soda, and make sure everyone in the car has a bottle of ice water. To make it more interesting, add sliced lemons, limes, or cucumber for a little flavor.*

- **Plan ahead.** *Review your road trip route in advance. In addition to packing low-carb snacks for the road, select spots along the way where you can stop and eat. Find other interesting locations where everyone can get out and stretch their legs and maybe even fit in a quick walk to make up for all of the hours sitting in the car.*

- **Eat frequently.** *Try to have a healthy meal or low-carb snack every two to three hours. This will help keep your hunger in check and make it a lot easier to resist the foods that might get you off track. Pack some snacks, and make sure you have plenty of ice if you're bringing a cooler to keep refrigerated items well chilled.*

- **At a convenience store:** *Convenience stores can be a little too convenient with it comes to sugary fountain drinks, cookies and crackers, and chips. Calm your cravings with a bag of nuts, such as almonds or cashews, or even sunflower seeds, the quintessential road trip snack. Jerky is always an option, although check the label, because some brands are higher in sugar than others. Many convenience stores sell hard-boiled eggs, which make for an easy protein-packed snack, or even packages of single-serve pickles and olives, plus vacuum-packed tuna packets, cheese sticks, mozzarella, and prosciutto roll-ups.*

- **At a fast-food restaurant:** *Sometimes the drive-through is the only option. See page 145 for the best low-carb choices at fast-food restaurants.*

Low-Carb Road Trip Snacks
- Sliced vegetables with cream cheese
- String cheese; cheese slices or cubes
- Hard-boiled or deviled eggs
- Olives
- Beef or turkey jerky (cured without sugar)
- Berries
- Pickles
- Pork rinds
- Celery sticks stuffed with peanut butter
- Portable tuna packets

How to Keep Moving on the Road
- If you're on vacation and engaging in activities such as hiking, swimming, skiing, windsurfing, or even just walking while taking in the sights, chances are you're getting plenty of exercise.
- If you're spending most of your waking hours in a conference room or driving from one appointment to another, you'll probably want to find a way to get in some physical activity. Here are some ways to do so:
  - Do a quick workout in your hotel's fitness center.
  - Put on your walking or running shoes and get out and explore your surroundings.
  - Pack a set of resistance bands in your suitcase so you can work out in your hotel room, plus add in some core exercises and plyometrics.

Low-Carb Swaps for Your Salty and Sweet Cravings

If you want to skip the restaurant (and save a little money), here are some delicious low-carb swaps for some of your favorite foods that you can make at home:

- **French fries and potato chips:** *Try Cheesy Cauliflower Bites on page 249.*
- **Wings:** *Try Crispy Cajun Chicken Thighs with Celery Ranch Salad on page 231.*
- **Nachos:** *Try "Nachos" Stuffed Chicken Breast on page 236.*
- **Cookies and brownies:** *Try Flourless Salted Peanut Butter Chocolate Chip Cookies on page 274 or Chocolate-Hazelnut Brownie Bites on page 275.*
- **Ice cream:** *Try No-Churn Mint Chip Ice Cream on page 270 or Fresh Peach and Cinnamon No-Churn Ice Cream on page 279.*

There's a world of delicious food out there, and with Atkins 100, you can enjoy most of it while still making healthy choices!

CHAPTER 7

BUDGET-FRIENDLY AND ENVIRONMENT-FRIENDLY HACKS FOR LOW-CARB LIVING

If you keep good food in your fridge, you will eat good food.
—*Unknown*

WHO DOESN'T LOVE TO EAT OUT or take advantage of food delivery apps at your fingertips with the meals arriving in minutes or a quick trip through the drive-through? I've shown you my favorite hacks for making the best choices while eating out, but although those options are convenient, they can be a burden on your budget, and since you can't control the quality of the ingredients or portion sizes, they aren't always the best for your healthy lifestyle. There's the notion that "eating healthy" is more time consuming and expensive, but it doesn't have to be that way at all! With some simple planning and smart shopping and cooking strategies, Atkins 100 can be a budget-friendly way of healthy eating. Even better? Not only is eating healthy food better for you (this should be a no-brainer at this point), it's also better for the environment. I'll show you why this is true, as well as give you some environmentally friendly tips for low-carb living, suggestions for plant-based meals, and options for including more veggies in every meal.

BUDGET-FRIENDLY HACKS FOR ATKINS 100

You've already discovered how important it is to plan your meals and stick to a shopping list, and cooking at home is also inherently easier on your wallet. Try my hacks for budget-friendly shopping and cooking:

....

Tip: When you plan ahead (both your meals and your shopping list), you'll waste less food and eliminate most last-minute trips to the store. You can also have your groceries delivered for a fee (your delivery driver is making multiple grocery drop-offs, which is also more efficient) or schedule a time to pick them up while you're already out and about doing errands.

....

Buy fewer processed foods. Some foods are way cheaper in their less-processed form. For example, a block of cheese is cheaper than shredded cheese; dried beans are cheaper than canned beans. Whole grains such as brown rice and oats are cheaper per serving than most processed cereals. Less-processed foods are also often sold in larger quantities and give you more servings per package.

Stop buying junk food. By now it should be no surprise to you that soda, crackers, and cookies provide little in the way of nutrition and are packed with unhealthy ingredients. They are also expensive. When you skip the foods filled with high-glycemic carbs and sugar, you can use more of your budget for higher-quality, healthy foods.

Stock up during sales. If you have favorite products or staples that you use frequently, stock up on them when they're on sale. Just make sure that they will last for a while and won't expire in the meantime or that they will freeze well.

Shop the canned foods aisle. Fill your pantry with cans of tomatoes, green chilies, and chipotle and adobo peppers, plus cans of fiber-rich beans if dried beans aren't available. Jars of banana peppers, sun-dried tomatoes, and artichoke hearts will add flavor to your recipes. And don't forget to freshen up your dried herb and spice supply. Turn to page 89 for a quick refresher on stocking your low-carb pantry.

Buy cheaper cuts of meat. Fresh meat can be a little pricey; however, you can find many cuts of meat that cost much less. Beef tenderloin is a wonderfully tasty cut of meat (with a price tag to match), but cuts such as chuck and sirloin contain more marbling (streaks of fat that run throughout the meat), which makes them superflavorful, tender, and juicy. They're best suited to slow cooking, so think stews, soups, roasts, and braises. Inexpensive cuts of pork, such as tenderloin, rib chops, shoulder, and butt are very tasty when properly prepared. With a little planning and a slow cooker or Instant Pot, you will have a delicious low-carb meal.

Buy a whole chicken. It's almost always less expensive than prepackaged chicken parts; if you learn to cut up your own chickens, you'll save money. You can also roast a whole chicken and use it for multiple meals and snacks throughout the week.

Get creative with fish. Go beyond salmon, halibut, shrimp, and scallops. Bluefish, catfish, tilapia, sardines, mackerel, and mussels are all less expensive choices.

Occasionally replace meat with other proteins. Eating less meat may be a good way to save money, and it may also be better for the environment (see page 168). Be good to your budget by replacing meat with other protein sources one or two days a week, such as eggs, canned fish (see page 204 for a delicious low-carb Mediterranean Tuna Salad), or legumes. You can prepare eggs in any number of ways (see page 112), while tofu and other soy foods can stand in for chicken and turkey. The freezer section of your grocery store may also have vegetarian protein crumbles, and you may find plant-based burgers and ground "beef" in the refrigerated meat section (see page 174 for more information)— they are a great alternative for ground beef and can transform into chili or tacos in no time. All these meatless protein options may cost less and are nutritious and easy to prepare.

Shop for produce in season. Local produce that is in season is generally cheaper, and it is also usually at its peak in both nutrients and flavor. Produce that is not in season has often been transported halfway around the world to get to your store, which is not good for either the environment or your budget. Also, buy produce by the bag if you can. That is usually a lot cheaper than buying by the piece. If you buy more than you need, you can freeze the rest or incorporate it into your low-carb meal plans the following week.

Skip the salad in a bag. Greens that have been washed, chopped, and sealed in a bag are far more expensive than those that are sold as individual heads.

Know that convenience can still be cost conscious. If time is in short supply, a salad in the bag, packaged spiralized zucchini, or prericed cauliflower and precooked rotisserie chicken will enable you to throw together a fast and easy low-carb meal (plus leftovers).

Buy frozen fruits and vegetables. Fresh fruits, berries, and vegetables are usually in season only a few months per year. Quick-frozen produce is usually just as nutritious. It is cheaper, available all year, and sometimes sold in large bags. Frozen produce is great to use when cooking, making smoothies, or as toppings for oatmeal or full-fat Greek yogurt. Furthermore, you gain the advantage of being able to take out only what you're about to use. The rest will be kept safe from spoiling in the freezer. Reducing your produce waste is also a great way to save money.

Buy in bulk. You'll find bulk nuts, seeds, beans, and grains at lower prices because you're not paying a premium for fancy packaging or marketing. You can also buy bulk amounts of meat, chicken, pork, lamb, and fish. When you get home from the store, portion the meat into individual or multiple servings and freeze.

Grow your own produce. If you can, it is a great idea to cultivate your green thumb and grow your own produce. Seeds are very cheap to buy. Lettuce and other salad greens, tomatoes, cucumbers, carrots, radishes, green beans, hot peppers, and zucchini, as well as herbs such as cilantro, oregano, sweet basil, and mint are all great options for beginning gardeners. Having a continuous supply of produce in season saves you money at the store. And if you've ever bitten into a juicy tomato picked at the peak of ripeness straight off the vine, you know how much better homegrown produce tastes compared with store-bought varieties.

If you don't have the space or talent to set up a full-blown vegetable garden, you can grow almost any vegetable, such as tomatoes, in a container, and you can grow herbs and greens in pots, hanging baskets, or a hydroponic garden system. You can even grow herbs indoor on a sunny windowsill.

Cook once, eat twice. Taking your own lunch to work or school and eating leftovers for dinner is an excellent way to control the quality and cost of your meals. Make the most of leftovers by cooking dishes that can do double duty as lunch the next day, or try one of the delicious lunch recipes starting on page 203. Don't forget about dinner! You can double a recipe so that you have dinner for one or two extra nights. Repurpose leftover vegetables by adding them to egg dishes or adding broth and some leftover chicken or meat to make a savory soup. If you have a little time on the weekend, you can roast a chicken or make a beef, pork, or lamb roast, then reap the benefit of all the delicious leftovers in salads, curries, stir-fries, stews, and soups.

Learn to love less expensive foods. You can't eat prime rib and lobster every day, can you? There are a lot of foods available that are inexpensive, healthy, and delicious. By getting a little creative and researching new low-carb recipes, whether in this book, at Atkins.com, or on Pinterest or Instagram, you can find new ways to use inexpensive staples such as eggs, beans, seeds, frozen vegetables and fruits, cheaper cuts of meat, and whole grains.

DIY your salad dressing. Save money on bottled salad dressing by whipping up your own fresh and flavorful batch with the Beyond Basic Vinaigrette recipe on page 112.

Be smart about snacks. Skip single-serving packages and buy almonds, pistachios, and other nuts in bulk. Repackage in a plastic zip bag for a grab-and-go snack you can throw into your purse, briefcase, or gym bag.

Keep a variety of oils on hand. Oils run the gamut when it comes to price and quality, so it's wise to use them accordingly. Buy larger containers of less expensive oils—canola oil, olive oil, peanut oil—to use for stir-frying and sautéing, and keep smaller containers of flavorful, high-quality, cold-pressed oils, such as extra-virgin olive oil, walnut oil, and hazelnut oil, to drizzle onto soups, salads, and veggies.

Stock up on stock. Chicken, beef, or vegetable broth or stock is the savory and naturally low-carb backbone of many low-carb slow cooker recipes, one-pot meals, and soups. Most unopened packaged or canned stock or broth will last up to a year in your pantry. Or you can make your own chicken, beef, or vegetable broth. It will stay fresh for up to three days in your refrigerator and up to three months in your freezer. Bone broth is also a nutrient-rich, flavorful addition to any recipe; you can also buy this in most supermarkets or make your own.

Avoid wasting food. According to the National Resources Defense Council, about 40 percent of the food produced in the United States is never eaten. If an item has a short shelf life (certain meats and produce), buy just what you need for two to three days so you can use it up before it goes bad. Or make sure you cook or freeze it before then. The longer the shelf life of a food, the more you can stock up on it, although there's a fine line between stocking up and hoarding. There's no need to over-buy, as you may lose track of all that you have stashed in your pantry and freezer.

Store Food as a Chef Does

Chefs have learned that storing food properly is key when it comes to not wasting food. Start by cleaning and prepping any food that needs it, as well as repackaging as necessary. Any meat that you don't plan to use within three days should be frozen.

Arrange perishables from the back of your fridge to the front, with leftover cooked items, less hardy fruits and vegetables and dairy products with the closest expiration dates front and center and less perishable items in the back.

You can store staples such as onions, potatoes, and other root vegetables; hard squashes such as butternut or acorn squash; apples; and citrus fruits in a cool, dark place such as the pantry.

Fresh herbs will last longer if you cut an inch off the bottom and store them standing up in fresh cold water in your fridge.

. . . .

Tip: Find a budget-minded buddy! It's natural to lose a little motivation here and there, making blowing your food budget on a few lunches or dinners out seem tempting. Gather some friends and/or family who are also on the budget bandwagon and exchange recipes and tips with them.

. . . .

THE SLOW COOKER: THE SECRET OF BUDGET-FRIENDLY LOW-CARB COOKING

There's nothing better than coming home to the savory smells of a rich, satisfying low-carb meal that has been simmering for hours. A slow cooker or Instant Pot is a lifesaver when it comes to whipping up budget-friendly low-carb meals.

Here are my tips for successful low-carb slow cooking:

- **Keep the ingredients you need on hand.** Stock your freezer with chopped veggies and packages of ground beef, flank steak, chicken thighs and breast, and sausage, and fill your pantry with cans of diced tomatoes, chicken and beef stock, and spices.
- **Prep the night before.** Thaw out any frozen ingredients, cut and trim meat, chop vegetables, measure out dry ingredients, and prepare any sauce if necessary so all you have to do in the morning is add the ingredients to your slow cooker (reheat any sauce that you made before you add it). If your slow cooker has a removable insert, once you prep your ingredients, you can add them all to the insert, remove it from the slow cooker, and refrigerate it overnight. In the morning, bring the insert to room temperate for 30 minutes to an hour (while you're getting ready to go out), and then set the slow cooker to your desired time before you head out the door.
- **Boost the flavor.** Browning your meat and sautéing veggies pumps up the flavor of your low-carb slow cooker meal, and it's definitely worth the extra few minutes it takes to do this. Toward the end of the cooking time, you can add fresh herbs, lemon juice, lime juice, citrus zest, hot sauce, grated Parmesan, olive oil, sautéed garlic, shallots, or ginger to brighten the flavor of your dish.

There are many low-carb recipes that can be modified to cook in your slow cooker. Look for key words such as "braised" and "slow-roasted" and dishes such as soups, stews, and chili. These are all perfect for your slow cooker if you follow these tips:

- **Watch the amount of liquid.** Since a slow cooker stays covered the entire time your food is cooking, steam accumulates and any liquid that you add doesn't evaporate, meaning a dish that is supposed to thicken as it cooks may end up waterier when prepared in a slow cooker. Reduce the liquid by almost half if you're not using a slow cooker recipe. If the original recipe does not call for liquid, add ½ cup water or broth. If your dish is still a little too watery by the end of the cooking time, you can remove the lid to let the liquid reduce or remove the insert and finish on the stove top.

- **Time it right.** If the original cooking time for your recipe is about an hour, set your slow cooker to four to six hours on high. If the original cooking time for your recipe is more than an hour, you can set it for eight hours or more on low.

Mindful Eating: Five Reasons Why It's Better for Your Budget

We've all found ourselves mindlessly munching in front of the TV or computer, grabbing a doughnut from the office break room without even thinking about it, helping the kids "clean their plates," or stress eating just before a deadline. Yet studies suggest that eating more slowly and thoughtfully may help you make healthier food choices. This is called mindful eating, when you bring your full attention to the ritual of eating and enjoying the flavors and experience. Listening to your body's cues can help you learn when you're eating because you're actually hungry or purely out of habit or if you're bored or stressed out. Here's how you can go from eating mindlessly to eating mindfully:

1. **Write down your food consumption.** *I swear by keeping a food journal. It can help you understand what triggers and situations may cause you to overeat, and over time you can begin to understand these patterns. This is also a place where you can track your Net Carb intake, meals, and snacks. It also might help you think twice before you splurge on junk food or fast food to cure a temporary craving. You can go old school and write everything down on paper or download the free Atkins Weight Loss app.*

2. **Stay connected.** *If you haven't done so already, check out the community at Atkins.com, where you can learn and share tips for eating more mindfully while living a low-carb lifestyle.*

3. **Plan ahead.** *Temptations lurk everywhere when hunger hits if you haven't planned your low-carb meals and snacks for the day. Plus, regular meals and snacks will help keep your appetite satisfied, so you're less likely to mindlessly munch or divert to the drive-through.*

4. **Make your meals special.** *There's nothing special about eating dinner while you're standing at the counter sorting through your junk mail. Take a moment to set the table, light a candle, put away your electronics, and savor the flavors of your food; truly slow down and enjoy your meal.*

5. **Know when you've had enough.** *It takes your stomach about twenty minutes to send your brain a signal that it is full, which is why it's easy to overeat. If you're still hungry at the end of your meal, drink a big glass of water, go for a walk, or do the dishes and then see if your stomach is still growling.*

SUSTAINABLE EATING HABITS: GOOD FOR YOUR POCKETBOOK AND THE ENVIRONMENT

With Atkins 100, you're making conscious low-carb choices every day, but what and how you eat can also have a positive impact on the environment. While many of my budget-friendly hacks are also environmentally friendly (think less food waste), here are four more ways you can make sustainable food choices that go hand in hand with living a low-carb lifestyle:

• **Shop locally.** Support local farmers whenever you can, whether that means perusing your farmer's market for fresh veggies and fruit in season, swinging by a farm stand, or having your eggs, milk, and cheese delivered from a dairy near you and buying meat and poultry that has been raised locally and sustainably. When you shop locally and in season, it costs less and you are supporting your local economy; in addition, transporting fruits and vegetables around the country has a negative impact on the environment, as does growing fruits and vegetables in greenhouses.

- **Occasionally cut back on meat.** A juicy steak is delicious, but raising and transporting livestock require more energy and resources than does growing plants. Just one plant-based meal a day or a plant-based day of eating a week has a positive impact.
- **Support the organic food industry.** The regulations surrounding organic foods encourage sustainable farming practices, such as limiting the use of synthetic pesticides and controlling weeds and pests naturally. Animals are raised with plenty of access to the outdoors and are given organic, hormone-free feed, while diseases are prevented naturally.
- **Pass on plastic.** Invest in reusable grocery bags. You can even buy mesh cotton or nylon produce bags and skip the plastic ones on the roll. Swap out your aging plastic food storage containers for glass containers.

LOW-CARB MENUS AT HOME

Whether it's date night in, a farm-to-table evening, or Sunday brunch, we've put together some delicious menus featuring our brand-new low-carb recipes that are good for your budget, perfect for omnivores, and heavy on flavor and fresh vegetables:

SEAFOOD LOVERS
- Zucchini Fritters with Sun-dried Tomato Pesto (page 251)
- Lemon Baked Cod with Braised Cauliflower and Greens (page 243)

• Flourless Salted Peanut Butter Chocolate Chip Cookies (page 274)

FARM TO TABLE

• Peach Caprese Skewers (page 262)
• Seared Hanger Steak with Harissa Butter and Spinach (page 241)
• Berries with Lemon Cashew Cream (page 271)

A TASTE OF THE MEDITERRANEAN

• Mezze Plate with Falafel-Spiced Yogurt Dip (page 256)
• Roasted Salmon with Crushed Green Olive, Lemon, and Fennel Salad (page 226)
• Fresh Peach and Cinnamon No-Churn Ice Cream (page 279)

SUNDAY BRUNCH

• Tropical Green Smoothie (page 193)
• Hearty Greens and Mushroom Breakfast Scramble (page 185)
• "Zucchini Bread" Protein Pancakes (page 196)

A PLANT-BASED ATKINS 100 IS AN OPTION

Though vegetables contain some carbs, they are also a valuable source of nutrients and fiber. Replacing starchy or refined carbs (think potatoes, pasta, and rice) with veggies makes for a satisfying and colorful addition to your plate. A plant-based approach also has a favorable impact on the environment, as it takes far less time and expense to grow broccoli than it does a steak. Foods such as vegetables, fruits, legumes, nuts, and olive oil go hand in hand with plant-based meals. You can't go wrong when you fill up on Foundation Vegetables and low-glycemic fruits. Grains with a high fiber and protein content, such as oatmeal, bulgur, and buckwheat, slow the digestion of carbs and their path into your bloodstream. Now, this doesn't mean you have to give up meat entirely, but you'll love these tasty plant-based suggestions that will open up your nutritional palate to a whole new range of options that will add variety to your meals and snacks.

....

Tip: Though you don't have to become a full-blown vegetarian, it's quite possible to follow a plant-based eating approach while on Atkins 100 (see page 63).

....

Here's Why You Should Love Veggies!

1. **They help control your appetite.** *Thanks to the fiber and water in vegetables, they fill you up more efficiently than do processed carbs that are low in fiber.*

2. **They keep your energy levels at an even keel.** *The fiber in vegetables slows down the release of their carbohydrates, which can help regulate your blood sugar.*

3. **They pack a powerful nutritional punch.** *They tend to be low in calories, high in fiber, and rich in nutrients, which means you naturally consume fewer calories and still feel satisfied.*

4. **They contain important antioxidants.** *The carotenoids, flavonoids, phenols, and other antioxidants and phytonutrients in veggies help control the free-radical pathology caused by all the chemicals we are exposed to in the environment.*

5. **Their consumption is associated with a decreased risk of developing many diseases.** *The research on this topic is quite emphatic: increasing your consumption of vegetables will decrease your risk of developing the diseases that are the biggest killers of Americans. Whether it be heart disease, stroke, cancer or diabetes, large-scale epidemiological data show that eating more vegetables is protective.*

Low-Carb Science Bite

Do you spend a lot of time looking at electronic devices? They emit high-energy blue light that can ultimately affect your eyesight by causing oxidative damage to the central part of the retina, known as the macula. Interestingly, a lot of research shows that a certain carotenoid, lutein, accumulates in the macula and acts as a filter for blue light, protecting the eye from the damage caused by it. A higher intake of lutein has been linked to preventing or even improving both age-related macular degeneration (AMD) and cataracts. Foods high in lutein include—you guessed it—vegetables! Go for green leafy vegetables such as kale or spinach, as well as peppers and broccoli.

OPTIONS FOR ADDING MORE VEGGIES TO YOUR MEALS

BREAKFAST

- **Strengthen your smoothies.** A breakfast shake is an easy, tasty way to get more veggies into the start of your day. Add ½ cup frozen cauliflower rice, a cup of baby spinach or baby kale, an avocado, some cucumber or zucchini, or some canned pumpkin to your favorite smoothie to bulk up the veggies.
- **Create a veggie stack.** Start with a large slice or two of tomato or cooked sweet potato, layer on cubed cucumber, arugula, and thinly sliced green onion, add a drizzle of vinaigrette or creamy dressing, and top with an egg, breakfast sausage, Canadian bacon, or smoked salmon.
- **Boost your bread.** Add shredded zucchini to a low-carb banana bread or breakfast muffin recipe.

- **Love leftovers for breakfast.** Breakfast does not have to be just breakfast food. Last night's leftovers can make a satisfying and veggie-rich breakfast, too!
- **Go for eggs.** Bake an egg in half an avocado or half a bell pepper. Top with cheese and salsa for a breakfast fiesta!

LUNCH

- **Make a sandwich.** Roll up deli meat, cheese, and mayo around a veggie. Pickles, cucumber spears, asparagus, bell pepper slices, olives, zucchini spears, sprouts, avocado, and steamed green beans are some options to try.
- **Create a cauliflower rice taco bowl.** Start with a base of ¾ cup frozen cauliflower rice, top with frozen fajita veggies, and microwave until warm. Then top with your favorite salsa, guacamole, cheese, and leftover taco meat.
- **Make a veggie bowl.** Start with 1 cup frozen broccoli (or any frozen veggies you have on hand), add 1 tablespoon butter, microwave until hot, mix in shredded cheese, and top with slices of fully cooked warm sausage.
- **Make a portobello pizza.** Use a portobello mushroom cap as the base for a quick pizza by topping it with pizza sauce, mozzarella cheese, and some mini pepperoni. Pop it under the broiler to melt the cheese and enjoy!
- **Prepare a pasta bowl.** Use zucchini "noodles" as the base of a quick heat-and-eat "pasta" bowl. Top the zucchini with hot pasta sauce and grilled chicken.

DINNER

- **Swap pasta for veggie "noodles."** Fill half your plate with zucchini "noodles," then mix in some whole grain noodles for any pasta meal.
- **Get creative with "rice."** Replace half your rice with cauliflower rice for the best of both worlds.

- **Sneak veggies in.** "Hide" some vegetables in pasta sauce by adding a handful or two of baby spinach, kale, or shredded zucchini as it heats. You can add veggies to any sauce, not just pasta sauce.
- **Say "cheese."** Make a quick cheese sauce by melting cream cheese in heavy cream, then adding your choice of shredded cheese to flavor. Top any steamed or roasted veggie with cheese sauce, and watch it disappear!
- **Roast your veggies.** Toss broccoli, Brussels sprouts, or cauliflower with some melted butter and seasoning blend, and roast on a sheet pan at 425°F until the veggies begin to brown, about 25 minutes.
- **Break out your spiralizer.** Use a spiralizer to make noodles out of broccoli stems, zucchini, sweet potatoes, winter squash, or any other rigid vegetable. Use them in salads, soups, or veggie bowls to add texture and interest.

Small Changes Lead to Big Results!
Three plant-based meals per week in place of meat can save about:

- 225 square feet of land
- 120 gallons of water
- 54 miles of car emissions

Let's Talk About Plant-Based "Burgers"

If you love the taste of a juicy burger but want to limit your intake of animal products, "burgers" and "ground beef" products such as Impossible Burger and Beyond Burger are both vegan and *gluten free and use plant-based protein, usually from peas, beans, lentils, or soy; they also contain small amounts of fiber, as well as nutrients such as iron and vitamin B_{12} that vegan and vegetarian diets often lack.*

The Impossible Burger uses heme, soy, and potato protein and actually contains more iron than a beef burger and 6 grams of Net Carbs (without a bun). Heme is an essential molecule naturally found in plant and animals that causes the Impossible Burger to "bleed" like real meat when it's cooked. Both the heme and soy are made from genetically modified organisms (GMOs).

The Beyond Burger uses pea protein isolate, a powder made by extracting protein from yellow peas, and contains 2 grams of Net Carbs (without a bun). By comparison, a burger made from beef contains no carbs.

These two burgers cook, smell, and taste like real meat. Some people say if they had not been told that what they were eating wasn't a "real" burger, they might have never guessed. Keep in mind that even if you go with a plant-based burger, you're not doing anything good for your health if you serve it with a white flour bun and corn syrup–sweetened ketchup.

Read "Meat" Labels

There are other plant-based "meat" products on the market, but be sure to examine the ingredients list, as they may contain sugar or "natural" flavors (which could be anything), as well as other less-than-healthy additives.

What Are GMOs?

A genetically modified organism (GMO) is a plant, animal, microorganism, or other organism whose genetic makeup has been modified in a laboratory using genetic engineering. One of the biggest pros for developing GMO crops is pest resistance, which reduces the need for the wide-scale use of synthetic pesticides.

HOW TO MAKE YOUR MEALS PLANT BASED AND BUDGET FRIENDLY

Try these hacks for adding some plant-based love to your weekly meal:

- Roast some vegetables and pan-fry tofu. The method described in the Red Curry Tofu and Rainbow Chard Stew recipe on page 205 is excellent for making crispy tofu.
- Make a taco bowl with a base of cauliflower rice, meatless crumbles with taco seasoning, salsa, cheese, and guacamole.
- Use meatless chicken strips in an anchovy-free Caesar salad.
- Add meatless Italian meatballs to zucchini "noodles" and pasta sauce. Or add chopped tempeh to your favorite pasta sauce while it is warming.
- Wrap a grilled meatless "burger" patty in lettuce leaves and serve with a side salad and sweet potato oven fries.
- Sauté shredded cabbage and bell pepper strips with garlic, green onion, and ginger and serve over cauliflower rice with tofu and peanut sauce.

LOW-CARB PLANT-BASED MENUS

Whether you're vegetarian or vegan or you would just like to add more low-carb plant-based dishes to your meal plans, you can take your pick from these menus:

VEGAN FEAST

- Chili-Spiced Papaya (page 259)
- Red Curry Tofu and Rainbow Chard Stew (page 205)
- Berries with Lemon Cashew Cream (page 271)

VEGGIE LOVERS

- Cheesy Cauliflower Bites (page 249)
- Vegetarian Ramen Zoodle Bowls (page 227)
- No-Churn Mint Chip Ice Cream (page 270)

SOUP AND SALAD

- Coconut Curry Squash Soup (page 208)
- Moroccan Chicken Mason Jar Salad (substitute tempeh for chicken) (page 209)
- Creamy Coconut-Cocoa Ice Pops (page 269)

Are you ready to start cooking? One of the most budget-friendly things you can do is cook the majority of your meals at home. Flip to part three for your choice of low-carb breakfast, lunch, dinner, snack, and dessert recipes, which have been taste tested by the Atkins team. I promise that you will love them!

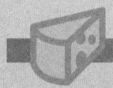

PART THREE

Mouthwatering Low-Carb Recipes for Optimal Energy and Flavor

RECIPES

CHAPTER 8

BREAKFASTS

Scrambles, Smoothies, Pancakes, and Prosciutto

WHAT BETTER WAY to start your day than with a savory (or sweet) and satisfying low-carb breakfast? Whether you're grabbing a nutrient-packed smoothie on the go or you have the time to prepare Sunday brunch and you're craving low-carb versions of bagels and lox or pancakes, these recipes fit the bill.

. . . .

Tip: Since it's easier to add an ingredient to a recipe than to subtract one, these recipes start at the Atkins 20 level of Net Carbs, with simple tips for leveling up to Atkins 40 and Atkins 100 with additions such as a side of sweet potato or swaps such as apples for blueberries.

. . . .

Tip: Many of these recipes use kosher salt, which is preferred over table salt. Kosher salt is less processed and contains fewer additives than table salt, and its coarse consistency and flat grain size make it ideal for sprinkling over vegetables and seasoning poultry, meat, and fish.

. . . .

....
Tip: *You can mix and match Atkins 20 or Atkins 40 recipes with Atkins 100 recipes if they sound more appealing to you. This way of eating is truly personalized!*
....

GREEN SHAKSHUKA

SERVES 4 • TIME: *Active*—20 minutes *Total*—35 minutes

This popular Israeli breakfast dish gets a satisfying, delicious, green spin with Swiss chard and zucchini standing in for higher-carb tomatoes and bell peppers. An excellent source of antioxidants, chard also provides ample potassium, calcium, and magnesium, all of which help maintain a healthy blood pressure. Choose green or rainbow chard, as you like. Both work well in this recipe.

> *2 tablespoons olive oil*
> *1½ large bunches Swiss chard (about 1 pound), stems and leaves coarsely chopped and kept separate (7 packed cups)*
> *1 large zucchini, cut into ¼-inch-thick half moons (2 cups)*
> *2 garlic cloves, finely chopped*
> *Kosher salt*
> *⅓ cup vegetable broth*
> *1 teaspoon ground cumin*
> *½ teaspoon smoked paprika*
> *¼ teaspoon red pepper flakes, plus more for garnish*
> *8 large eggs*
> *4 ounces feta cheese, crumbled (about 1 cup)*
> *2 tablespoons chopped cilantro (optional)*

1. Heat the oil in a 10- to 12-inch skillet over medium-high heat. Add the chard stems, zucchini, garlic, and ¾ teaspoon salt; cook, stirring

occasionally, until softened, about 5 minutes. Add the chard leaves, vegetable broth, cumin, paprika, and red pepper flakes. Continue cooking until the chard is tender, about 2 minutes.

2. Reduce the heat to medium-low. Using the back of a wooden spoon, create eight 2-inch depressions in the chard mixture. Crack an egg into each. Season the eggs with a pinch of salt. Cook until the whites are close to set, 6 to 8 minutes. Sprinkle the cheese over the top, then cover and cook until the whites are set and the yolks are cooked to your liking, 2 to 5 minutes more.

3. Top with the cilantro and red pepper flakes, if desired. Use about ¾ cup of greens with 2 eggs and 1 ounce of cheese for each serving.

PER SERVING

ATKINS 20 • Net Carbs: 8 grams; Total Carbs: 11 grams; Fiber: 3 grams; Protein: 19 grams; Fat: 22 grams; Calories: 316; FV: 4

ATKINS 40 *with 1 serving Cauliflower Rice with Butter and Chives (recipe follows) per serving* • Net Carbs: 11 grams; Total Carbs: 16 grams; Fiber: 5 grams; Protein: 22 grams; Fat: 29 grams; Calories: 394; FV: 6

ATKINS 100 *with ¼ cup cooked quinoa per serving* • Net Carbs: 17 grams; Total Carbs: 21 grams; Fiber: 4 grams; Protein: 21 grams; Fat: 23 grams; Calories: 371; FV: 4

....

Tip: *"FV" refers to the number of grams of Net Carbs that come from Foundation Vegetables on the Acceptable Foods list (see page 94).*

....

CAULIFLOWER RICE WITH BUTTER AND CHIVES

SERVES 4 • TIME: *Active*—10 minutes *Total*—10 minutes

Any soft herb you have on hand or in your garden works well in this flavorful veggie "rice." Try basil, mint, parsley, and/or dill in place of or with the chives.

······························

Tip: *If you prefer to purchase frozen or fresh prericed cauliflower rather than make your own, use 1 pound prericed cauliflower.*

······························

1 medium head cauliflower (about 1 pound), stem and florets coarsely chopped, or 1 pound frozen prericed cauliflower, not thawed

2 tablespoons unsalted butter

½ teaspoon kosher salt

¼ teaspoon freshly ground black pepper

2 tablespoons finely chopped chives or scallion

1. If you're starting with a head of cauliflower, pulse half of the chopped florets in a food processor until it resembles rice. Transfer to a 10- to 12-inch skillet. Repeat with the remaining cauliflower.

2. Add the butter, salt, and pepper to the skillet. Cook over medium-high heat until the cauliflower is tender, about 5 minutes. Remove from the heat and stir in the chives or scallions. Serve warm.

3. If you're using prericed cauliflower, cook it according to the package instructions. In a 10- to 12-inch skillet, melt the butter, salt, pepper, and chives or scallions over medium heat, swirling the skillet once or twice, 1 to 2 minutes. Add the cooked cauliflower and cook, stirring, just to combine, about 1 minute more. Serve warm, a generous ¾ cup per person.

PER SERVING

Net Carbs: 2 grams; Total Carbs: 5 grams; Fiber: 3 grams; Protein: 2 grams; Fat: 6 grams; Calories: 80; FV: 2

HEARTY GREENS AND MUSHROOM BREAKFAST SCRAMBLE

SERVES 4 • TIME: *Active*—40 minutes *Total*—40 minutes

Power up your morning with this veggie-packed scramble, which is finished with plenty of melted cheese and fiber-rich, heart-healthy avocado. At the market, look for cremini mushrooms (also known as baby portobellos), which have a deeper, more complex flavor than the white button variety. Resist the urge to stir the mushrooms as they cook! Letting them caramelize undisturbed in sizzling butter gives them a gorgeous, deep-golden sear. For an ultracreamy soft scramble, take the skillet off the flame before the eggs are fully set. They'll finish cooking off the heat in a matter of seconds, while maintaining a creamy center.

....

Tip: *Yellow or white cheddar can be used. Choose whichever type and level of sharpness you prefer.*

....

Tip: *Any hearty greens, such as Swiss chard, escarole, spinach, and the like, can be used in place of kale.*

....

8 large eggs
¼ cup heavy cream
Kosher salt
Freshly ground black pepper
2 tablespoons unsalted butter
8 ounces crimini mushrooms, thinly sliced (about 3 cups)
3 scallions, thinly sliced, divided (scant ½ cup)
2 cups finely chopped lacinato kale leaves and tender stems or other hearty greens (from about 3 large leaves)

1 cup shredded sharp cheddar cheese (4 ounces)
1 medium avocado, thinly sliced, for garnish

1. In a large bowl, whisk together the eggs, cream, ½ teaspoon salt, and ¼ teaspoon pepper. Set aside.
2. In a 10- to 12-inch nonstick skillet, melt the butter over medium-high heat. Stir in the mushrooms and half of the scallions. Cook, undisturbed, until the mushrooms are golden, 7 to 9 minutes.
3. Stir in the kale, ¼ teaspoon salt, and ¼ teaspoon pepper; reduce the heat to medium, and cook until the kale begins to soften, about 1 minute, then stir in the eggs. Using a rubber spatula, stir the eggs around and across the skillet until fluffy and barely set, about 3 minutes. Stir in the cheese and take the skillet from the heat. Continue stirring until the cheese is melted and the eggs are just set, about 1 minute more.
4. Divide the scramble among four serving plates, about 1 heaping cup of scramble each. Top with the avocado and remaining scallions. Serve warm.

PER SERVING

ATKINS 20 • Net Carbs: 8 grams; Total Carbs: 12 grams; Fiber: 4 grams; Protein: 23 grams; Fat: 35 grams; Calories: 440; FV: 1

ATKINS 40 *with 1 low-carb tortilla per serving* • Net Carbs: 12 grams; Total Carbs: 31 grams; Fiber: 19 grams; Protein: 28 grams; Fat: 38 grams; Calories: 510; FV: 1

ATKINS 100 *with 1 Siete almond flour grain-free tortilla per serving* • Net Carbs: 16 grams; Total Carbs: 22 grams; Fiber: 6 grams; Protein: 26 grams; Fat: 40.5 grams; Calories: 540; FV: 1

SMOKED SALMON STACK

SERVES 4 • TIME: *Active*—25 minutes *Total*—25 minutes

This mile-high salmon stack recalls the classic bagel and lox, but unlike its carb-laden counterpart, it won't weigh you down. Each bite is packed with the flavors of the NYC favorite: fresh dill, crunchy cucumber, smoked salmon, and briny capers, with a dollop of sour cream standing in for cream cheese. Heart-healthy smoked salmon delivers protein, filling fats, and plenty of omega-3s. Make this deceptively easy dish for yourself or for a brunch with friends.

....

Tip: More tender and slightly milder in flavor than adult kale, baby kale is often sold in clear clamshell boxes alongside other packaged lettuce greens. If you can't find baby kale, chopped mature kale can also be used.

....

1 tablespoon plus 1 teaspoon olive oil

4 large eggs

Kosher salt

Freshly ground black pepper

½ cup sour cream

1 English cucumber, cut into ¼-inch cubes (about 2 ¼ cups or 10 ounces)

2 tablespoons coarsely chopped dill

8 ounces smoked salmon

¼ cup thinly sliced scallion (1 scallion)

4 teaspoons drained capers, patted dry

4 cups loosely packed baby kale (2 ounces)

1½ teaspoons fresh lemon juice, plus wedges for serving

1. In a large nonstick skillet, heat 1 tablespoon of oil over medium-high heat. Add the eggs one at a time. Cook until the edges are golden, the whites are set, and the yolks are still runny, about 3 minutes.

(The eggs can be flipped and cooked longer to be more well done, if desired.) Take the skillet from the heat. Season with salt and pepper.

2. Dollop 2 tablespoons of sour cream in the center of each of four serving plates. Top with a heaping ½ cup cucumber, ½ tablespoon dill, and a pinch of salt in a tight round single layer, then stack 2 ounces salmon, 1 egg, 1 tablespoon scallion, and 1 teaspoon capers on top. If you are adding Sweet Potato Toast for Atkins 40 (see recipe below), make it the base on top of the sour cream, then stack the dill, salmon, and remaining ingredients on top. Use the cucumber in the salad.

3. In a bowl, toss together the kale, lemon juice, a pinch each of salt and pepper, and the remaining teaspoon of oil. Mound 1 cup of salad alongside each of the salmon stacks and serve with the lemon wedges.

PER SERVING

ATKINS 20 • Net Carbs: 5 grams; Total Carbs: 7 grams; Fiber: 2 grams; Protein: 19 grams; Fat: 17 grams; Calories: 254; FV: 2

ATKINS 40 *with 1 "slice" Sweet Potato Toast (recipe follows)* • Net Carbs: 9 grams; Total Carbs: 12 grams; Fiber: 3 grams; Protein: 19 grams; Fat: 18 grams; Calories: 288; FV: 6

Atkins 100 *with 1 slice Ezekiel sprouted grain bread per serving* • Net Carbs: 17 grams; Total Carbs: 22 grams; Fiber: 5 grams; Protein: 23 grams; Fat: 18 grams; Calories: 334; FV: 2

SWEET POTATO TOAST

SERVES 4

1 teaspoon olive oil

1 medium sweet potato, cut into four ¼-inch-thick rounds (about 4 ounces uncooked)

Salt

Pepper

In a large nonstick skillet, heat the oil over medium-high heat until hot but not smoking. Add the sweet potato rounds. Reduce the heat to medium-low. Season the rounds with a generous pinch each of salt and pepper and cook until the bottoms are golden, 1 to 2 minutes. Reduce the heat to low, flip the potato rounds, season with salt and pepper, cover, and cook until tender, about 1 to 2 minutes more. Serve warm or at room temperature.

PER SERVING

Net Carbs: 5 grams; Total Carbs: 6 grams; Fiber: 1 gram; Protein: 1 gram;
Fat: 1 gram; Calories: 34; FV: 5

ONE-SKILLET MEXICAN BREAKFAST

SERVES 4 • TIME: *Active*—35 minutes *Total*—35 minutes

Tempeh, a plant-based protein most often made from soybeans, is packed with nutrients, fiber, and antioxidants and is less processed than other meat alternatives. It's also fermented, which makes it easily digestible and gives it a savory umami flavor that's appealing to meat eaters and vegetarians alike. Here it's finely chopped (which helps it meld with the lime juice and spices and cook quickly) and topped with fried eggs, zesty salsa, and creamy avocado.

....
Tip: *Look for tempeh next to tofu in the refrigerated case at your grocery store. Ground chicken, beef, or turkey can be used instead, if you like.*
....

¼ cup olive oil, divided
1 medium zucchini, chopped
1 garlic clove, finely chopped
8 ounces tempeh, finely chopped
1 teaspoon chili powder

¾ *teaspoon ground cumin*
½ *teaspoon garlic powder*
Cayenne pepper
2 tablespoons fresh lime juice
Kosher salt
6 ounces baby spinach or coarsely chopped whole leaves (5 packed cups)
8 large eggs
4 tablespoons chopped cilantro, for garnish
4 tablespoons jarred salsa, for garnish
1 medium avocado, halved, pitted, and thinly sliced, for garnish

1. In a large nonstick skillet, heat 2 tablespoons of oil over medium-high heat. Add the zucchini and garlic. Cook, stirring occasionally, until golden, about 5 minutes. Add the tempeh, chili powder, cumin, garlic powder, a pinch of cayenne pepper, lime juice, ¾ teaspoon salt, and 1 tablespoon water and stir to combine. Cook until the flavors are blended, about 3 minutes, then stir in the spinach and cook until wilted, about 1 minute more. Remove from the heat. Cover to keep warm.
2. In a large nonstick skillet, heat 1 tablespoon of oil over medium-high heat. Crack in 4 eggs and cook until the whites are crisp at the edges and set around the yolk, about 2 minutes.
3. Transfer the cooked eggs to a plate. Repeat with the remaining eggs.
4. Divide the tempeh mixture among four bowls, about 1 cup in each. Top each portion with 2 fried eggs, 1 tablespoon cilantro, 1 tablespoon salsa, and ¼ of the avocado.

PER SERVING

ATKINS 20 • Net Carbs: 8 grams; Total Carbs: 16 grams; Fiber: 8 grams; Protein: 25 grams; Fat: 29 grams; Calories: 439; FV: 2

ATKINS 40 with 1 serving Cauliflower Rice with Butter and Chives (see page 183) per serving • Net Carbs: 11 grams; Total Carbs: 21 grams; Fiber: 10 grams; Protein: 27 grams; Fat: 36 grams; Calories: 517; FV: 4

ATKINS 100 *with ¼ cup cooked brown rice per serving* • Net Carbs: 20 grams; Total Carbs: 29 grams; Fiber: 9 grams; Protein: 27 grams; Fat: 30 grams; Calories: 499; FV: 2

SPICY SAUSAGE PATTIES WITH CAULIFLOWER HASH BROWNS

SERVES 4 • TIME: *Active—*50 minutes *Total—*50 minutes

These spicy, herb-packed sausage patties come with a side of crispy cauliflower hash browns, making them healthier and more flavorful than anything you'll find at a diner. To yield crispy golden florets that are tender on the inside, you'll steam the florets before sautéeing them in butter and smoky spices. A final flurry of grated Parmesan coats each floret in salt-kissed cheesy goodness.

Tip: *For milder-tasting hash browns, use sweet paprika instead of smoked and omit the cayenne pepper.*

For the Cauliflower Hash Browns
3 cups coarsely chopped cauliflower florets (from 1 medium head)
2 tablespoons unsalted butter
1 tablespoon olive oil
½ teaspoon kosher salt
¼ teaspoon smoked paprika
Cayenne pepper
1 tablespoon grated Parmesan cheese

For the Spicy Sausage Patties
1 pound ground pork
4 scallions, thinly sliced (generous ½ cup)
½ cup chopped cilantro (leaves and stems)

2 tablespoons no-sugar sriracha, plus more for serving

Kosher salt

3 tablespoons olive oil

1 tablespoon chopped parsley, for garnish

....

Tip: Look for brands of sriracha with no added sugar.

....

1. Prepare the Cauliflower Hash Browns: In a large skillet, combine the cauliflower and ⅓ cup water. Cover and cook over medium-high heat until tender, about 5 minutes. Pour off any leftover liquid. Return the skillet to medium-high heat. Stir in the butter, oil, salt, paprika, and a pinch of cayenne pepper, then spread the cauliflower into a single layer. Cook until golden and crispy, about 4 minutes per side, then stir in the cheese and transfer to a plate; loosely cover with foil to keep warm. Wipe out the skillet.

2. Prepare the Spicy Sausage Patties: In a large bowl, mix together the pork, scallions, cilantro, sriracha, and ¾ teaspoon salt. Form the mixture into 12 patties, about 2 inches in diameter and ¼ inch thick. In the same skillet, heat 1 tablespoon of oil over medium heat. Working in batches of four, cook the patties until golden and cooked through and an instant-read thermometer inserted into the thickest part registers 145°F, about 3 minutes per side.

3. Serve 3 warm sausage patties with ½ cup cauliflower hash browns and topped with ¾ teaspoon parsley. Pass the sriracha at the table.

PER SERVING

ATKINS 20 • Net Carbs: 6 grams; Total Carbs: 9 grams; Fiber: 3 grams;
Protein: 24 grams; Fat: 37 grams; Calories: 459; FV: 3

ATKINS 40 with ½ slice of Ezekiel sprouted grain bread per serving
• Net Carbs: 11 grams; Total Carbs: 16 grams; Fiber: 5 grams;
Protein: 25 grams; Fat: 38 grams; Calories: 499; FV: 3

ATKINS 100 *with 1 slice of Ezekiel sprouted grain bread per serving* •
Net Carbs: 18 grams; Total Carbs: 24 grams; Fiber: 6 grams; Protein:
28 grams; Fat: 28 grams; Calories: 539; FV: 3

TROPICAL GREEN SMOOTHIE

SERVES 4 • TIME: *Active*—10 minutes *Total*—10 minutes
Makes four 16-ounce drinks

Frozen bananas are often used in smoothies to give them a creamy consistency. Here, heart-healthy avocado and a can of coconut milk provide the same creamy richness with fewer carbs. If you're new to kale or haven't yet been convinced, this smoothie is a great place to start—you reap all its nutritional benefits (including fiber, vitamins, and brain-boosting phytonutrients) while enjoying the flavor of the greens balanced by vanilla, coconut, avocado, and tangy lime juice.

....
*Tip: To transform this protein-packed breakfast into
a smoothie bowl, simply add less water.*
....
*Tip: To extend the shelf life of flaxseeds and chia seeds, store
them in the refrigerator or freezer.*
....

1 medium avocado, halved and pitted
4 servings vanilla-flavored whey protein powder
2 cups ice
*2 cups packed baby kale or roughly chopped kale leaves (stems
    removed) (3 ounces)*
2 tablespoons ground flaxseeds
2 tablespoons chia seeds
1 (15-ounce) can unsweetened full-fat coconut milk

4 tablespoons fresh lime juice
1 tablespoon unsweetened coconut flakes, for garnish

Scoop the flesh of half of the avocado into a blender. Add half of the protein powder, ice, kale, flaxseeds, chia seeds, coconut milk, 1 cup water, and 2 tablespoons lime juice. Puree until smooth. Thin the mixture with water if you prefer a less thick smoothie. Divide among two 16-ounce glasses, repeat with the remaining ingredients, top with coconut flakes, and serve.

PER SERVING

ATKINS 20 • Net Carbs: 8 grams; Total Carbs: 16 grams; Fiber: 8 grams;
    Protein: 35 grams; Fat: 33 grams; Calories: 486; FV: 0

ATKINS 40 *with ¼ cup fresh raspberries added per serving* • Net Carbs: 10
    grams; Total Carbs: 20 grams; Fiber: 10 grams; Protein: 33 grams;
    Fat: 33 grams; Calories: 501; FV: 0

ATKINS 100 *with ½ cup fresh pineapple chunks added per serving* •
    Net Carbs: 18 grams; Total Carbs: 27 grams; Fiber: 9 grams;
    Protein: 35 grams; Fat: 33 Calories: 527; FV: 0

"MEXICAN HOT CHOCOLATE" SMOOTHIE

SERVES 4 • TIME: *Active*—10 minutes *Total*—10 minutes
Makes four 16-ounce drinks

Thanks to chocolate-flavored protein powder, warming spices such as cinnamon and nutmeg, and a pinch of cayenne pepper, this smoothie boasts all the decadent flavors of Mexican hot chocolate—and it's packed with veggies, too. Frozen cauliflower not only supercharges this smoothie with fiber, immune-boosting vitamin C, anti-inflammatory compounds, and antioxidants, it also makes it übercreamy, and its neutral flavor doesn't distract from the other ingredients.

....
Tip: Cacao nibs, which are made from crushed cocoa beans, have a bitter, chocolatey flavor and are rich in antioxidants.
....

1 medium avocado, halved and pitted

1¼ cups frozen riced cauliflower

4 cups unsweetened almond milk

2 cups ice

3 servings chocolate-flavored whey protein powder

1 serving vanilla-flavored whey protein powder

1 packed cup fresh baby spinach or chopped spinach leaves

2 tablespoons chia seeds

2 teaspoons ground cinnamon

¼ teaspoon ground nutmeg

Cayenne pepper

4 teaspoons cacao nibs, for garnish

Scoop the flesh of half of the avocado into a blender. Add half of the cauliflower, almond milk, ice, protein powders, spinach, chia seeds, cinnamon, nutmeg, and a pinch of cayenne pepper. Puree until smooth, then divide between two glasses. Repeat with the remaining ingredients. Top the smoothies with cacao nibs and serve.

PER SERVING

ATKINS 20 • Net Carbs: 9 grams; Total Carbs: 18 grams; Fiber: 9 grams; Protein: 29 grams; Fat: 13 grams; Calories: 314; FV: 2

ATKINS 40 *with ¼ cup fresh strawberry halves added per serving* • Net Carbs: 11.5 grams; Total Carbs: 21 grams; Fiber: 9.5 grams; Protein: 30 grams; Fat: 13 grams; Calories: 326; FV: 2

ATKINS 100 *with ½ frozen banana added per serving* • Net Carbs: 22 grams; Total Carbs: 32 grams; Fiber: 10 grams; Protein: 30 grams; Fat: 13 grams; Calories: 366; FV: 2

"ZUCCHINI BREAD" PROTEIN PANCAKES

SERVES 4 • TIME: *Active*—40 minutes *Total*—40 minutes

The high-glycemic carbohydrates in a slice of zucchini bread or stack of buttermilk pancakes are likely to leave you feeling a late-afternoon energy slump—and craving more sugar. A far more nutritious and equally delicious alternative? These tender, fluffy pancakes, made with a low-carb flour mix, which boast all the warming flavors of zucchini bread while keeping your energy level balanced. These pancakes freeze well, so you can double the recipe to keep a stash on hand. Thaw them overnight in the fridge, then gently reheat in the microwave.

> **Tip:** *When shopping for zucchini, look for medium to small ones, vibrant in color and with a bit of stem attached. They are more tender and less fibrous than larger ones.*

⅔ pound small to medium zucchini (2 to 3, depending on size)
4 tablespoons unsalted butter
½ cup unsweetened almond milk
2 large eggs, lightly beaten
2 tablespoons sugar-free pancake syrup
1 cup Atkins Flour Mix (see recipe following)
2 teaspoons baking powder
1½ teaspoons cinnamon
¼ teaspoon nutmeg
¼ teaspoon kosher salt

1. Into a large bowl, coarsely grate the zucchini (you should have 1¼ packed cups. Save any additional zucchini for another use). Melt 2 tablespoons of the butter. Add the butter, almond milk, eggs, and syrup to the bowl with the zucchini; stir to combine.

2. In a second large bowl, whisk together the flour mix, baking powder, cinnamon, nutmeg, and salt; add the dry ingredients to the zucchini mixture and stir just to combine (do not overmix).

3. In a large nonstick skillet, melt ½ tablespoon of the remaining butter over medium heat and swirl to coat. Working in batches, pour the batter into the skillet in scant ¼ cupfuls. Cook the pancakes until the bottoms are golden brown and bubbles form at the top, about 3 minutes. Flip and cook until cooked through and the other side of the pancake is golden brown, about 2 minutes more.

4. Divide the pancakes (about 3 per person) among four plates and serve.

PER SERVING

ATKINS 20 • Net Carbs: 7 grams; Total Carbs: 18 grams; Fiber: 11 grams; Protein: 34 grams; Fat: 15 grams; Calories: 310; FV: 1

ATKINS 40 *with ¼ cup fresh blueberries per serving* • Net Carbs: 12 grams; Total Carbs: 24 grams; Fiber: 12 grams; Protein: 35 grams; Fat: 15 grams; Calories: 332; FV: 1

ATKINS 100 *with ½ baked apple per serving* • Net Carbs: 17 grams; Total Carbs: 30 grams; Fiber: 13 grams; Protein: 35 grams; Fat: 15 grams; Calories: 356; FV: 1

ATKINS FLOUR MIX

MAKES ABOUT 3 CUPS

¼ cup wheat bran

1⅛ cups whole grain soy flour

⅔ cup vanilla-flavored or unflavored whey protein powder

¼ cup organic 100% whole ground golden flaxseed meal

⅔ cup wheat gluten

In a large bowl, combine all the ingredients and mix thoroughly. Use immediately or store in an airtight container in the refrigerator for up to 1 month.

PER SERVING

Net Carbs: 4.9 grams; Total Carbs: 8 grams; Fiber: 3 grams; Protein: 19 grams; Fat: 4 grams; Calories: 140; FV: 0

BROCCOLINI AND BACON EGG BITES

SERVES 4 • TIME: *Active*—20 minutes *Total*—45 minutes

These creamy, tender, grab-and-go egg bites are inspired by the Starbucks favorite but are steamed using a simple water bath method rather than a more complicated sous vide technique. Think of broccolini as broccoli's younger cousin—it's mellower in flavor, and the florets get extra-crispy when sautéed. These egg bites reheat well, so you can make a big batch over the weekend and enjoy them for breakfast or a protein-packed snack all week long. To heat, simply microwave for 15 seconds, flip, and microwave 10 seconds more. Special equipment: You'll need a standard regular muffin tin and nonstick cupcake liners, or a nonstick muffin tin, or silicone egg-bite molds, which you can find at kitchen shops and online. Makes 8 egg bites.

. . . .

*Tip: For a vegetarian version, omit the bacon and use
1 tablespoon olive oil in place of the bacon fat.*

. . . .

*Nonstick cooking spray
5 slices no-sugar-added bacon (4 ounces)
Kosher salt
5 large eggs*

3 ounces cream cheese

2 tablespoons feta cheese

1 tablespoon hot sauce (such as Cholula)

4½ ounces broccolini (5 to 7 stalks), stalks and florets thinly sliced

1½ cups baby arugula

1 tablespoon lemon juice

1 tablespoon extra-virgin olive oil

Freshly ground black pepper

1. Preheat the oven to 350°F. Lightly coat eight silicone egg-bite mold cups or eight cups of a standard nonstick muffin tin with cooking spray, or line a regular (not nonstick) muffin tin with nonstick muffin liners and set into a large baking pan.

2. In a large nonstick skillet, cook the bacon over medium heat until golden, about 5 minutes per side. Transfer to a paper towel–lined plate to drain. Chop the bacon into small pieces.

3. Meanwhile, in a blender, puree the eggs, cream cheese, feta cheese, hot sauce, and ¼ teaspoon salt until smooth.

4. Pour off all but 1 tablespoon of fat from the skillet. Add the broccolini, 1 tablespoon water, and ¼ teaspoon salt. Cook over medium-high heat, stirring frequently, until the broccolini is tender, 3 to 5 minutes. Remove from the heat.

5. Fill each of the egg cups with 1 heaping teaspoon of bacon and 1 heaping tablespoon of broccolini. Top with the egg mixture, filling the cups to about ⅛ inch from the top (you may have a bit left over; discard or sauté in a skillet for a mini snack). Add just enough boiled water to the baking pan(s) to come halfway up the sides of the molds.

6. Bake the egg bites until set, 20 to 25 minutes. Take the pan(s) from the oven, then take the molds from the water bath(s). Let the egg bites cool for a few minutes, then remove them from the molds.

7. In a medium bowl, toss together the arugula, lemon juice, oil, and a pinch each of salt and pepper. Place ¾ cup of salad and 2 egg bites on each of four plates and serve.

PER SERVING

ATKINS 20 • Net Carbs: 5 grams; Total Carbs: 6 grams; Fiber: 1 gram; Protein: 13 grams; Fat: 33 grams; Calories: 380; FV: 1

ATKINS 40 *with ¼ cup fresh blueberries per serving* • Net Carbs: 9 grams; Total Carbs: 11 grams; Fiber: 2 grams; Protein: 14 grams; Fat: 34 grams; Calories: 400; FV: 1

ATKINS 100 *with 1 slice of Eziekel sprouted grain bread per serving* • Net Carbs: 22 grams; Total Carbs: 28 grams; Fiber: 6 grams; Protein: 19 grams; Fat: 34 grams; Calories: 499; FV: 1

WARM ESCAROLE WITH EGGS AND PROSCIUTTO (AKA ITALIAN-STYLE BACON AND EGGS)

SERVES 4 • TIME: *Active*—30 minutes *Total*—30 minutes

This thirty-minute breakfast is everything you crave from a morning meal: crispy fried eggs, a bit of salty prosciutto, a sprinkling of cheese, and some feel-good greens. Escarole, a vitamin-rich member of the chicory family that is commonly used in Italian cuisine, tastes slightly bitter when eaten raw, but sautéeing it mellows its bite. A pinch of crushed red pepper flakes and lemon zest add bold flavor to every bite.

....

Tip: Spinach, frisée, or even Boston lettuce can be used in place of the escarole, if desired.

....

2 tablespoons plus 4 teaspoons extra-virgin olive oil
6 cups coarsely chopped escarole (from a scant 1-pound head)

¼ *teaspoon red pepper flakes*
¼ *teaspoon grated lemon zest*
8 *large eggs*
8 *slices (about 4 ounces) prosciutto*
¼ *cup grated Parmigiano-Reggiano cheese*
Kosher salt

1. In a large skillet, heat 2 tablespoons of oil over medium-high heat. Add half of the escarole and the red pepper flakes. Cook until slightly wilted, then add the remaining escarole and lemon zest. Cook, stirring occasionally, until wilted, about 5 minutes. Transfer the escarole to a bowl.

2. Wipe the skillet dry and heat 2 tablespoons of oil over medium heat. Cook 4 eggs, undisturbed, until the whites are set, the edges are golden, and the yolks are still runny, 4 to 5 minutes. Season with a pinch of salt. Transfer to a plate and repeat with the remaining oil and eggs.

3. Arrange ½ cup escarole, 2 eggs, and 2 slices prosciutto on each of four plates. Sprinkle each plate with 1 tablespoon of cheese and more red pepper flakes, if desired. Season with salt to taste and serve.

PER SERVING

ATKINS 20 • Net Carbs: 2 grams; Total Carbs: 4 grams; Fiber: 2 grams; Protein: 23 grams; Fat: 25 grams; Calories: 340; FV: 0

ATKINS 40 *with 2 ounces baked sweet potato per serving* • Net Carbs: 12 grams; Total Carbs: 16 grams; Fiber: 4 grams; Protein: 24 grams; Fat: 25 grams; Calories: 390; FV: 10

ATKINS 100 *with 3 ounces baked sweet potato per serving* • Net Carbs: 18 grams; Total Carbs: 22 grams; Fiber: 4 grams; Protein: 24 grams; Fat: 25 grams; Calories: 415; FV: 15

RECIPES

CHAPTER 9

LUNCHES

Salads, Soups, Stews, and Sandwiches

COLORFUL, NUTRIENT-RICH vegetables are the "foundation" of these vibrant low-carb lunch dishes, while fresh herbs and spices add huge pops of flavor. You can whip up an elevated version of a budget-friendly tuna salad, indulge in the comforting flavors of pho, or satisfy your appetite with a protein-packed lunch bowl.

....

Tip: *As with the breakfast recipes, these recipes start at the Atkins 20 level of Net Carbs, with simple tips for leveling up to Atkins 40 and Atkins 100 with additions such as brown rice or rice noodles for the bowls.*

....

Tip: *With Atkins 100, you can mix and match Atkins 20 or Atkins 40 recipes if they sound more appealing to you. This way of eating is truly personalized!*

....

MEDITERRANEAN TUNA SALAD

SERVES 4 • TIME: *Active*—30 minutes *Total*—30 minutes

This colorful tuna salad is composed mostly of pantry ingredients. Paprika and cayenne pepper lend mild spice, while lemon juice and fresh herbs brighten things up. Store-bought marinated artichoke hearts add complexity with little fuss. Tuna is a nutritional powerhouse, filled with omega-3 fatty acids, potassium, and iron. Serve this salad over greens for a feel-good, protein-packed lunch.

....

Tip: Marinated artichoke hearts are sold jarred at most good grocers.

....

Tip: Buying blocks of feta cheese (rather than crumbles) gives you the flexibility to crumble or slice the cheese to any size you like.

....

4 (5-ounce) cans oil-packed tuna, drained
1 (6.5-ounce) jar quartered and marinated artichoke hearts
   (about 7), drained and coarsely chopped (¾ cup)
½ cup finely chopped packed fresh flat-leaf parsley
½ cup mayonnaise
3 tablespoons capers, rinsed, drained, and coarsely chopped
1 tablespoon grated lemon zest
2 tablespoons fresh lemon juice
½ teaspoon kosher salt
½ teaspoon paprika
¼ teaspoon freshly ground black pepper
Cayenne pepper
8 packed cups mixed greens (8 ounces)

4 ounces feta cheese, crumbled (1 cup) or sliced
Lemon wedges, for garnish

1. In a large bowl, use a fork to flake the tuna into large pieces. Add the artichoke hearts, parsley, mayonnaise, capers, lemon zest and juice, salt, paprika, black pepper, and a pinch of cayenne pepper. Gently stir to combine.
2. Arrange 2 cups mixed greens on each of four plates. Top each with about 1 cup of tuna salad and 1 ounce of cheese. Serve with lemon wedges.

PER SERVING

ATKINS 20 • Net Carbs: 7 grams; Total Carbs: 11 grams; Fiber: 4 grams; Protein: 38 grams; Fat: 39 grams; Calories: 564; FV: 3

ATKINS 40 *with 1 Mission Carb Balance flour tortilla per serving* • Net Carbs: 10 grams; Total Carbs: 29 grams; Fiber: 19 grams; Protein: 44 grams; Fat: 42 grams; Calories: 633; FV: 3

ATKINS 100 *with 1 slice of toasted Ezekiel sprouted grain bread per serving* • Net Carbs: 19 grams; Total Carbs: 26 grams; Fiber: 7 grams; Protein: 43 grams; Fat: 40 grams; Calories: 644; FV: 3

RED CURRY TOFU AND RAINBOW CHARD STEW

SERVES 4 • TIME: *Active*—40 minutes *Total*—40 minutes

Red curry paste and coconut milk lend warm spice and richness to this comforting vegan dish. Leftovers thicken in the refrigerator; loosen them with a splash of water or broth.

Tip: *This stew is medium spicy. For a mild spice level, reduce the curry paste to 1 tablespoon.*

....

Tip: *Pressing tofu between paper towels before cooking helps remove moisture, allowing for better crisping. To save time, start the tofu dressing first, then prep the remaining ingredients.*

....

Tip: *One pound of cubed skinless, boneless chicken or large peeled and deveined shrimp can be used in place of the tofu, if you prefer. Reduce the salt to ⅛ teaspoon and cook your protein of choice, stirring occasionally, until just cooked through (3 to 4 minutes for shrimp; 5 to 8 minutes for chicken), then adjust the salt to taste.*

....

16 ounces extra-firm tofu, drained and cut into ½-inch cubes

3 tablespoons olive oil

½ bunch rainbow chard (about 6 ounces), stems trimmed and chopped into bite-size pieces (¾ cup), leaves finely chopped (3 packed cups)

3 tablespoons finely chopped onion

2 tablespoons red curry paste

1 garlic clove, finely chopped

1 tablespoon peeled and finely chopped fresh ginger (from a 1-inch piece)

Kosher salt

Freshly ground black pepper

3 cups coarsely chopped cauliflower florets

1 (15-ounce) can unsweetened full-fat coconut milk, well stirred

1 cup vegetable broth

Unsweetened toasted coconut and chopped cilantro, for garnish

1. Arrange the tofu on a paper towel–lined plate or cutting board. Top with a few layers of paper towel and a heavy skillet. Let stand for 15 minutes to remove as much moisture as possible.

2. In a medium saucepan, heat 1 tablespoon of oil over medium-high heat. Add the chard stems and onion and cook, stirring occasionally, until just softened, about 5 minutes. Add the curry paste, garlic, ginger, ½ teaspoon salt, and a generous pinch of pepper and cook, stirring, until fragrant, about 1 minute.

3. Stir in the cauliflower, coconut milk, broth, and ½ teaspoon salt and bring to a simmer. Cover, reduce the heat to low, and simmer until the cauliflower is tender, 6 to 8 minutes. Remove the stew from the heat, stir in the chard leaves, and cover to keep warm.

4. Meanwhile, season the pressed tofu with ½ teaspoon of salt. In a large nonstick skillet, heat 2 tablespoons of oil over medium-high heat. Add the tofu and cook, undisturbed, until the underside is deep golden and crispy, about 5 minutes. Turn and continue cooking until the tofu is crispy all over, 3 to 4 minutes more.

5. Season the stew with salt to taste. Ladle 1¼ cups of soup into each of four bowls and top each equally with the tofu, coconut, and cilantro.

PER SERVING

ATKINS 20 • Net Carbs: 8 grams; Total Carbs: 12 grams; Fiber: 4 grams; Protein: 17 grams; Fat: 19 grams; Calories: 279; FV: 5

ATKINS 40 *with 1 tablespoon rinsed and drained canned chickpeas per serving* • Net Carbs: 10 grams; Total Carbs: 14 grams; Fiber: 4 grams; Protein: 18 grams; Fat: 19 grams; Calories: 290; FV: 5

ATKINS 100 *with 3 tablespoons rinsed and drained canned chickpeas per serving* • Net Carbs: 13 grams; Total Carbs: 18 grams; Fiber: 5 grams; Protein: 18 grams; Fat: 20 grams; Calories: 320; FV: 5

COCONUT CURRY SQUASH SOUP

SERVES 4 • TIME: *Active*—20 minutes *Total*—45 minutes

Fresh ginger lends antioxidants and anti-inflammatory properties to this bold, flavorful soup, and coconut milk is the key to its creamy consistency. Save a little to swirl on top for an impressive final touch.

....

Tip: *For a vegan version, omit the fish sauce and use vegetable broth in place of chicken broth.*

....

Tip: *Coconut oil is high in saturated fat, but it also gives "good" HDL cholesterol a boost and is fine to use on a low-carb diet. Use it occasionally to get its benefits, but don't go overboard.*

....

1 tablespoon coconut oil
2 tablespoons chopped onion
2 garlic cloves, finely chopped
1 tablespoon grated fresh ginger
¾ teaspoon kosher salt
1 tablespoon yellow curry paste
4 cups chicken broth
4 cups coarsely chopped zucchini (1¼ pounds or about 2½ medium)
2 tablespoons fresh lime juice
1 tablespoon Asian fish sauce (such as nuoc mam)
1 (13.5-ounce) can unsweetened full-fat coconut milk
¼ cup coarsely chopped cilantro leaves

1. In a large, wide, heavy pot, heat the coconut oil over medium heat. Add the onion, garlic, ginger, and salt. Cook, stirring constantly, for 1 minute, then stir in the curry paste and continue cooking until

fragrant, about 1 minute more. Add the broth, scraping the bottom of the pot to release any stuck bits, then add the zucchini. Increase the heat to high and bring to a boil, then reduce to a gentle simmer. Cover and cook until the zucchini is tender, 10 to 15 minutes.

2. Remove the pot from the heat and stir in the lime juice, fish sauce, and all but 2 tablespoons coconut milk. Carefully transfer the mixture to a blender or use an immersion blender and puree until smooth. Adjust the salt to taste.

3. Ladle 2 cups of soup into each of four serving bowls. Drizzle the remaining coconut milk on top, sprinkle with cilantro, and serve.

PER SERVING

ATKINS 20 • Net Carbs: 8 grams; Total Carbs: 11 grams; Fiber: 2 grams; Protein: 12 grams; Fat: 28 grams; Calories: 322; FV: 2

ATKINS 40 *with ¼ cup cooked butternut squash per serving* • Net Carbs: 12 grams; Total Carbs: 16 grams; Fiber: 4 grams; Protein: 13 grams; Fat: 28 grams; Calories: 341; FV: 2

ATKINS 100 *with 1 cup cooked butternut squash per serving* • Net Carbs: 21 grams; Total Carbs: 29 grams; Fiber: 8 grams; Protein: 14 grams; Fat: 28 grams; Calories: 398; FV: 2

MOROCCAN CHICKEN MASON JAR SALAD

SERVES 4 • TIME: *Active—*25 minutes *Total—*25 minutes

Mason jar salads aren't just trendy, they're a great way to tote a salad to work or school. Layering the ingredients strategically—starting with the dressing on the bottom and finishing with the leafy greens on top—ensures that the greens don't get soggy as the salad sits. To cut down on prep time, use cooked leftover or rotisserie chicken. Prep all four jars in one go (it takes only fifteen minutes), then grab them for lunch throughout the week.

· ·

Tip: *For a spicier salad dressing, add an extra pinch*
of cayenne pepper.

· ·

Tip: *For a vegetarian version, use tofu or tempeh in*
place of chicken.

· ·

For the dressing
⅓ cup mayonnaise

2½ tablespoons fresh lemon juice

½ teaspoon ground cumin

¼ teaspoon kosher salt

¼ teaspoon smoked paprika

Cayenne pepper

For the salad
1 cup ¼-inch cubes cucumber

20 pitted green olives, coarsely chopped

1 cup shredded red cabbage

20 ounces ½-inch cubes cooked chicken (about 3½ cups)

4 ounces feta cheese, crumbled (1 cup)

1 large avocado, halved, pitted, and cubed

2 tablespoons fresh lemon juice

4 cups packed baby arugula

¾ teaspoon kosher salt

½ cup alfalfa sprouts

1. Prepare the dressing: In a small bowl, whisk together the mayonnaise, lemon juice, cumin, salt, paprika, and a pinch of cayenne pepper. Adjust the salt and cayenne pepper to taste.

2. Prepare the salad: Divide the dressing among four 16-ounce jars with lids, about 2 tablespoons per jar. In each jar, layer ¼ cup cucumber, 5 olives, ¼ cup cabbage, 1 scant cup chicken, ¼ cup feta, ¼ avocado, ½ tablespoon lemon juice, 1 cup arugula, a generous pinch of salt, and 2 tablespoons sprouts, gently packing down the ingredients as you go. (For Atkins 40, end the layering with the almonds; for Atkins 100, begin with the quinoa.) Seal the jars with the lids and refrigerate until ready to serve. Eat from the jar (after shaking) or pour into a bowl.

PER SERVING

ATKINS 20 • Net Carbs: 5 grams; Total Carbs: 9 grams; Fiber: 4 grams; Protein: 35 grams; Fat: 31 grams; Calories: 453; FV: 2

ATKINS 40 *with 2 tablespoons sliced almonds per serving* • Net Carbs: 6 grams; Total Carbs:12 grams; Fiber: 6 grams; Protein: 38 grams; Fat: 36 grams; Calories: 519; FV: 2

ATKINS 100 *with ½ cup cooked quinoa per serving* • Net Carbs: 15 grams; Total Carbs: 21 grams; Fiber: 6 grams; Protein: 38 grams; Fat: 32 grams; Calories: 519; FV: 2

SPINACH, ASPARAGUS, AND CHARRED SCALLION FRITTATA

SERVES 4 • TIME: *Active*—20 minutes *Total*—30 minutes

Quick, delicious, and easy to vary, frittatas are fantastic make-ahead dishes that travel well and can be reheated in a microwave or enjoyed at room temp. Try this for a weeknight dinner, then take leftovers to work or school the next day for a protein- and vegetable-rich lunch. This beauty is packed with fiber-rich asparagus and vitamin-dense spinach and scallions that are crispy on the outside but tender within. Adding cream to the eggs gives the finished dish its custardy texture.

. . . .

Tip: *Any tender herb, such as chives, dill, or parsley or a combination, can be used in place of basil.*

. . . .

9 *large eggs*

⅓ *cup heavy cream*

Kosher salt

¼ *teaspoon freshly ground black pepper*

3 *teaspoons olive oil*

4 *scallions, trimmed, cut in half lengthwise and crosswise*

¾ *pound asparagus, trimmed and cut into ½-inch lengths (generous 2 cups)*

2 *cups packed baby spinach (3 ounces)*

⅓ *cup thinly sliced basil leaves, plus whole leaves for garnish*

⅓ *cup grated Parmesan cheese*

1. Set an oven rack in the upper third position. Preheat the oven to 400°F. In a large bowl, beat together the eggs, cream, ¾ teaspoon salt, and pepper. Set aside.

2. In a large nonstick ovenproof skillet, heat 1 teaspoon oil over medium-high heat. Add the scallions and cook until golden, turning once, about 2 minutes. Transfer to a plate.

3. Add the asparagus, ¼ teaspoon salt, and 2 teaspoons oil to the skillet. Cook until the asparagus is tender and lightly golden, about 5 minutes. Add the spinach and cook until wilted, about 1 minute more. Pour in the egg mixture and add the basil. Cook for 1 minute, then sprinkle the reserved scallions over the top.

4. Bake in the oven until the frittata is set, 8 to 10 minutes. Slide onto a cutting board and cut into 4 wedges. Top with cheese and basil leaves. Serve one wedge per person, warm or at room temperature.

PER SERVING

ATKINS 20 • Net Carbs: 6 grams; Total Carbs: 9 grams; Fiber: 3 grams;
   Protein: 20 grams; Fat: 24 grams; Calories: 334; FV: 3

ATKINS 40 *with ¼ cup fresh blueberries per serving* • Net Carbs: 10 grams;
   Total Carbs: 14 grams; Fiber: 4 grams; Protein: 20 grams; Fat: 24 grams;
   Calories: 354; FV: 3

ATKINS 100 *with 1 slice Ezekiel sprouted bread per serving* • Net Carbs:
   18 grams; Total Carbs: 24 grams; Fiber: 6 grams; Protein: 24 grams;
   Fat: 25 grams; Calories: 414; FV: 3

EASY CHICKEN PHO

SERVES 6 • TIME: *Active*—40 minutes *Total*—40 minutes

Traditional versions of pho, a Vietnamese dish consisting of rice noodles, thinly sliced beef, spiced beef broth, and a flurry of fresh herbs, can take more than a day to make—the longer the stock simmers, the more complex it becomes. This version uses smart shortcuts to make the recipe doable on a weeknight without skimping on flavor. Toasting fresh ginger, scallions, and aromatic spices before infusing store-bought broth with them results in a rich, slow-simmered flavor. If you're entertaining guests, set out small bowls with each of the garnishes and let everyone assemble their own bowl.

....

Tip: Shirataki noodles, brand name Miracle Noodles, are a low-calorie, zero-carb noodle alternative made from glucomannan, a type of fiber that comes from the root of the konjac plant. Look for them near the tofu in the refrigerator case at your grocery store.

....

1 (3- to 4-inch) knob fresh ginger, thinly sliced crosswise
4 scallions, trimmed, cut in half crosswise, whites and dark green
   parts separated

1 tablespoon whole black peppercorns

1 tablespoon whole cardamom pods

1 tablespoon whole coriander

4 pods whole star anise

2 cinnamon sticks

2 quarts chicken broth

1½ pounds boneless, skinless chicken breasts, quartered

12 ounces shirataki Miracle Noodles, rinsed and drained

3½ cups thinly sliced bok choy (about 4 baby bok choy or
    1 large head)

1 tablespoon soy sauce

3 tablespoons Asian fish sauce (such as nuoc mam)

Toppings

½ cup cilantro

½ cup mung bean sprouts

1 large jalapeño pepper, thinly sliced (½ cup)

1 lime, cut into 4 wedges

No-sugar sriracha

1. Using the back of a chef's knife, bruise the ginger slices. Heat a large, wide, heavy-bottomed pot over medium-high heat. Dry toast the ginger and scallion whites in the pot, turning occasionally, until golden and fragrant, about 4 minutes. Add the peppercorns, cardamom, coriander, star anise, and cinnamon sticks. Toast the spices, stirring constantly, 30 seconds more.

2. Add the broth, chicken, and 2 cups of water. Bring just to a boil, then reduce to a gentle simmer. Cover and cook until the chicken is cooked through, 8 to 10 minutes. Meanwhile, thinly slice the scallion greens and set them aside.

3. Remove the pot from the heat. Transfer the chicken to a cutting board and use a fork to shred it into small pieces.

4. Strain the broth into a large bowl; discard the solids. Return the broth to the pot and bring to a simmer. Add the noodles, bok choy, chicken, soy sauce, and fish sauce and cook until the bok choy is tender, about 3 minutes.

5. Ladle 3 cups of hot soup into each of four bowls and top with the scallion greens and the remaining toppings.

PER SERVING

ATKINS 20 • Net Carbs: 6 grams; Total Carbs: 11 grams; Fiber: 5 grams; Protein: 42 grams; Fat: 5 grams; Calories: 272; FV: 1

ATKINS 40 *with 2 tablespoons chopped dry roasted peanuts per serving* • Net Carbs: 9 grams; Total Carbs: 15 grams; Fiber: 6 grams; Protein: 45 grams; Fat: 14 grams; Calories: 371; FV: 1

ATKINS 100 *with ¼ cup cooked rice noodles per serving* • Net Carbs: 17 grams; Total Carbs: 22 grams; Fiber: 5 grams; Protein: 41 grams; Fat: 5 grams; Calories: 312; FV: 1

MUFFALETTA "HERO"

SERVES 4 • TIME: *Active—25 minutes Total—25 minutes*

This lightened-up version of the classic New Orleans muffaletta sandwich replaces carb-heavy bread with crunchy, vitamin-rich romaine lettuce. It's as fun to make as it is to eat. You'll roll up the tasty filling in the lettuce leaves, using parchment paper to both help roll and hold the sandwich. Slice and enjoy right away, or tote it to school, work, or a picnic.

....

Tip: Use the outer four leaves (the largest and most flexible) from three heads of romaine. Save the inner leaves to make salads. Iceberg lettuce can be substituted, using 6 to 8 leaves per sandwich.

....

. . . .

Tip: *Purchase pitted green olives for ease, or gently but firmly crush unpitted olives with the flat side of a chef's knife to easily remove the pits.*

. . . .

Tip: *For Atkins 40, the tortilla can be used as part of the roll-up or eaten on the side.*

. . . .

Tip: *For Atkins 100, the bread can be enjoyed on the side, or it could be used to make an open-faced sandwich instead of a roll-up.*

. . . .

16 large romaine lettuce leaves (about 8 ounces total), ends trimmed
12 ounces thinly sliced genoa salami
8 ounces thinly sliced provolone cheese (8 slices)
4 tablespoons mayonnaise
⅔ cup chopped roasted red peppers (from a jar)
1 cup pepperoncini peppers, thinly sliced
¾ cup pitted green olives, coarsely chopped

1. If the romaine leaves are longer than 10 inches, trim to a 10-inch length.

2. For each sandwich, place four romaine leaves, overlapping by 1 inch, in the center of a 12-by-12-inch sheet of parchment paper.

3. Place 3 ounces of salami over the romaine. Cover with 2 ounces of provolone, then spread with 1 tablespoon mayonnaise. Top with 2 tablespoons red peppers, 2 tablespoons pepperoncinis, and 1½ tablespoons olives.

4. Using parchment paper as a guide, roll up the lettuce as tightly as you can, tucking in the ends like a burrito about halfway through.

5. Twist the ends of the paper tightly to secure. Repeat to make the remaining three sandwiches.

6. When ready to eat, leaving the sandwich rolled in the parchment paper, use a sharp or serrated knife to cut the sandwich in half.

PER SERVING

ATKINS 20 • Net Carbs: 6 grams; Total Carbs: 7 grams; Fiber: 1 gram; Protein: 33 grams; Fat: 49 grams; Calories: 596; FV: 0

ATKINS 40 *with 1 Mission Carb Balance tortilla per serving* • Net Carbs: 10 grams; Total Carbs: 26 grams; Fiber: 16 grams; Protein: 38 grams; Fat: 52 grams; Calories: 666; FV: 0

ATKINS 100 *with 1 slice Ezekiel sprouted grain bread per serving* • Net Carbs: 18 grams; Total Carbs: 22 grams; Fiber: 4 grams; Protein: 37 grams; Fat: 49 grams; Calories: 676; FV: 0

TUSCAN SEARED STEAK AND SHREDDED KALE SALAD

SERVES 4 • TIME: *Active—*20 minutes *Total—*20 minutes

Leftover steak quickly turns into a superfood salad. Brussels sprouts and kale are packed with vitamins, fiber, and anti-inflammatory nutrients. These hardy greens hold up well even when dressed, so this is a great evening make-ahead to take to school or work the next day.

Tip: *To save time, look for shredded Brussels sprouts and grated Parmesan cheese at your grocery store.*

Tip: *Massaging cruciferous greens such as kale and Brussels sprouts softens their tough leaves and reduces their bitterness.*

⅓ cup freshly grated plus 2 ounces shaved Parmigiano-Reggiano
  cheese (about ⅓ cup shavings)
⅓ cup extra-virgin olive oil
1 teaspoon grated lemon zest
¼ cup fresh lemon juice
1 small garlic clove, grated or finely chopped
Kosher salt
Freshly ground black pepper
½ pound Brussels sprouts, trimmed
3 cups coarsely chopped lacinato kale leaves and tender stems
1½ pounds cooked steak, thinly sliced

1. Prepare the dressing: In a small bowl, whisk together the grated
   cheese, oil, lemon zest, lemon juice, garlic, a pinch of salt, and a generous pinch of pepper until smooth.
2. In the bowl of a food processor, pulse the Brussels sprouts until shredded. Transfer to a large bowl. Repeat with the kale, then add it to the
   sprouts. (The greens can be thinly sliced by hand if you don't have a
   food processor.)
3. Add ½ teaspoon of salt to the greens, then, using clean hands, mas-
   sage them for 1 minute to soften. Add the dressing and toss to combine. Adjust the seasoning to taste.
4. Divide the salad among four serving plates, about 1 cup on each.
   Top each with 6 ounces of steak and 1 heaping tablespoon of shaved
   cheese and serve.

PER SERVING

ATKINS 20 • Net Carbs: 5 grams; Total Carbs: 7 grams; Fiber: 2 grams; Protein:
  57 grams; Fat: 45 grams; Calories: 670; FV: 4

ATKINS 40 *with ¼ fresh apple per serving* • Net Carbs: 10.5 grams; Total
  Carbs: 13.5 grams; Fiber: 3 grams; Protein: 57 grams; Fat: 45 grams;
  Calories: 695; FV: 4

ATKINS 100 *with ½ fresh pear per serving* • Net Carbs: 17 grams; Total Carbs: 21 grams; Fiber: 5 grams; Protein: 57 grams; Fat: 45 grams; Calories: 721; FV: 4

CHIPOTLE TURKEY BOWLS WITH SPICY LIME DRESSING

SERVES 4 • TIME: *Active—*40 minutes *Total—*40 minutes

Canned chipotle peppers and a squeeze of fresh lime add vibrant and slightly smoky notes to this satisfying salady bowl. The creamy dressing tastes just like the classic taco favorite—without the added sugar and sodium.

....

Tip: Bok choy is a type of Chinese cabbage that ranks extremely high on the aggregate nutrient density index, meaning it delivers impressive levels of nutrients per calorie.

....

Tip: For a milder dish, you can adjust the amount of chipotle pepper in adobo sauce to your taste in both the dressing and the bowls.

....

Tip: A ripe avocado yields slightly when gently pressed. To ripen an avocado quickly, place it in a closed brown paper bag with a ripe banana. Ripe bananas release ethylene, which triggers ripening in other fruit.

....

For the dressing
⅓ *cup sour cream*
1½ *tablespoons fresh lime juice*
2 *teaspoons sauce from the chipotle pepper in adobo sauce can*

For the bowls
1 *tablespoon olive oil*

1½ pounds ground turkey

2 garlic cloves, minced

1 large head bok choy (about ¾ pound), trimmed, thinly sliced
(about 3½ cups)

3 tablespoons fresh lime juice

2 tablespoons seeded, finely chopped chipotle pepper in adobo sauce
(from a can)

Kosher salt

2 cups thinly sliced kale

1 avocado, halved, pitted, and cubed

½ cup chopped red bell pepper

¼ cup sliced pickled jalapeño peppers (from a can)

2 tablespoons chopped cilantro

Lime wedges, for garnish

1. Prepare the dressing: In a small bowl, stir together the sour cream, lime juice, chipotle in adobo sauce, and ¼ teaspoon salt until smooth.
2. Prepare the bowls: In a 10- to 12-inch skillet, heat the oil over medium-high heat. Add the turkey and garlic and cook, stirring with a wooden spoon to break up the meat, for 3 minutes. Add the bok choy, lime juice, chipotle pepper in adobo sauce, and 1 teaspoon salt. Continue cooking until the turkey is cooked through and most of the liquid has evaporated or been absorbed, about 5 minutes more. Remove from the heat.
3. Place ½ cup kale in each of four bowls. Top each with 1¼ cups of the turkey mixture, ¼ of the avocado, 2 tablespoons bell pepper, 1 tablespoon jalapeño, and ½ tablespoon cilantro. Drizzle with the dressing and serve with lime wedges on the side.

PER SERVING

ATKINS 20 • Net Carbs: 6 grams; Total Carbs: 12 grams; Fiber: 6 grams; Protein: 37 grams; Fat: 26 grams; Calories: 415; FV: 3

ATKINS 40 *with 1 serving of Cauliflower Rice with Butter and Chives (see page
183) per serving* • Net Carbs: 9 grams; Total Carbs: 17 grams; Fiber: 8
grams; Protein: 39 grams; Fat: 32 grams; Calories: 493; FV: 5

ATKINS 100 *with ¼ cup cooked brown rice per serving* • Net Carbs: 18 grams;
Total Carbs: 24 grams; Fiber: 6 grams; Protein: 39 grams; Fat: 26 grams;
Calories: 474; FV: 3

VIETNAMESE SHRIMP AND VEGETABLE NOODLE BOWLS

SERVES 4 • TIME: *Active—50* minutes *Total—50* minutes

Spiralized cucumber and crunchy sliced romaine lettuce take over for
rice noodles in this snappy, simple lunch bowl. The mildly spicy citrus-
sesame dressing gives the dish a traditional Vietnamese flair.

. . . .

*Tip: Frozen shrimp are great to keep on hand for quick, easy meals.
Thawing takes just a few minutes: place the shrimp in a colander
and hold under cool running water. Pat dry before cooking.*

. . . .

*Tip: Toasted sesame oil is pressed from toasted sesame seeds,
while regular sesame oil is pressed from untoasted seeds.
The former is richer in flavor but also sensitive to high-heat
cooking. Use it for dressings, marinades, and drizzling over
finished dishes. Use regular sesame oil, which can withstand
high heat, for cooking.*

. . . .

For the dressing
    4 tablespoons fresh lime juice
    3 tablespoons toasted sesame oil
    3 tablespoons hot water
    2 tablespoons fish sauce

 1 teaspoon granulated erythritol
 ¼ teaspoon of red pepper flakes
 2 garlic cloves, minced

For the bowls
 2 cups (½-inch) broccoli florets
 1 tablespoon olive oil
 1½ pounds peeled and deveined shrimp
 Kosher salt
 4 cups thinly sliced romaine lettuce
 1 medium cucumber, spiralized
 ½ cup mung bean sprouts
 ⅓ cup thinly sliced basil
 ¼ cup thinly sliced mint
 Lime wedges, for garnish

1. Prepare the dressing: In a small bowl, whisk together all of the ingredients.
2. Prepare the bowls: Bring a medium pot of salted water to a boil. Add the broccoli and cook until bright green and tender, about 3 minutes. Drain and set aside.
3. In a large skillet, heat the oil over medium-high heat. Pat the shrimp dry, season with a pinch of salt, and cook in an even layer, in batches if necessary, until opaque and cooked through, about 2 minutes per side.
4. Place 1 cup of the lettuce and about ¾ cup cucumber noodles into each of four serving bowls. Top with a quarter each of the shrimp, broccoli, sprouts, basil, and mint. Drizzle each with 3 tablespoons of the dressing and serve with lime wedges.

PER SERVING

ATKINS 20 • Net Carbs: 8 grams; Total Carbs: 11 grams; Fiber: 3 grams;
Protein: 26 grams; Fat: 16 grams; Calories: 282; FV: 2

ATKINS 40 *with 2 tablespoons chopped salted peanuts per serving* •
Net Carbs: 10 grams; Total Carbs: 14 grams; Fiber: 4 grams;
Protein: 32 grams; Fat: 25 grams; Calories: 389; FV: 2

ATKINS 100 *with ¼ cup cooked rice noodles per serving* • Net Carbs:
18 grams; Total Carbs: 21 grams; Fiber: 3 grams; Protein: 27 grams;
Fat: 16 grams; Calories: 330; FV: 2

RECIPES

CHAPTER 10

DINNERS

Main Meals for Every Occasion

DINNER IS A DELICIOUS home-cooked affair with these recipes, whether you want a meal in minutes, a hearty steak, or a feast worth lingering over. You'll find a plethora of international flavors that are sure to satisfy any appetite.

....

Tip: You can level up to Atkins 40 and Atkins 100 with easy additions such as sweet potato fries or even a minibaguette.

....

Tip: You can mix and match Atkins 20 or Atkins 40 recipes with Atkins 100 recipes if they sound more appealing to you. This way of eating is truly personalized!

....

ROASTED SALMON WITH CRUSHED GREEN OLIVE, LEMON, AND FENNEL SALAD

SERVES 4 • TIME: *Active*—30 minutes *Total*—30 minutes

Quick-cooking, heart-healthy salmon fillets are packed with omega-3 fatty acids, which have been shown to reduce blood pressure and inflammation. Here, lemon adds bright citrus flavor to both the fish and the crisp olive, lemon, and fennel salad that goes alongside.

Tip: If purchasing olives with pits in, you'll need 5 ounces.
If the olives are pitted, you'll need 3½ ounces.

Tip: Both skin-on and skinless salmon fillets work well here.
Use whichever you prefer or looks best at the market.

3 tablespoons olive oil, plus more for oiling the baking sheet
2 lemons
4 (6- to 8-ounce) salmon fillets
Kosher salt
Freshly ground black pepper
1 small fennel bulb, preferably with fronds
1 cup pitted Castelvetrano or Cerignola olives, crushed
1 tablespoon finely chopped shallot or red onion

1. Preheat the oven to 425°F. Line a baking sheet with foil and lightly grease with oil. Grate 1 tablespoon of zest from one of the lemons, then squeeze 2 tablespoons of juice from the same lemon; set aside. Thinly slice the remaining lemon into rounds. Remove and discard any seeds.

2. Season the salmon all over with ¾ teaspoon salt and ¼ teaspoon pepper. Place skin side down on the prepared baking sheet. Arrange the

lemon slices on top, then drizzle with 1 tablespoon oil. Roast until the fish is opaque and just cooked through (an instant-read thermometer inserted into the thickest part will register 145°F), 10 to 15 minutes, depending on the thickness.

3. Meanwhile, trim, core, and thinly slice the fennel bulb, then finely chop enough of the fronds, if available, to yield ¼ cup, or use as much as you have. In a bowl, toss together the fennel, fennel fronds, olives, shallot, lemon zest, lemon juice, ½ teaspoon salt, ¼ teaspoon pepper, and 2 tablespoons oil. Adjust the seasoning to taste.

4. Divide the salmon among four serving plates. Mound a heaping ¾ cup of the salad alongside each fillet and serve.

PER SERVING

ATKINS 20 • Net Carbs: 5 grams; Total Carbs: 8 grams; Fiber: 3 grams;
   Protein: 35 grams; Fat: 22 grams; Calories: 371; FV: 2

ATKINS 40 *with 2 tablespoons chopped toasted walnuts per serving* • Net
   Carbs: 5 grams; Total Carbs: 9 grams; Fiber: 4 grams; Protein: 37 grams;
   Fat: 33 grams; Calories: 475; FV: 2

ATKINS 100 *with ½ cup steamed parsnips per serving* • Net Carbs: 16 grams;
   Total Carbs: 21 grams; Fiber: 5 grams; Protein: 36 grams; Fat: 23 grams;
   Calories: 434; FV: 13

VEGETARIAN RAMEN ZOODLE BOWLS

SERVES 4 • TIME: *Active*—30 minutes *Total*—30 minutes

This quick, vibrant one-pot ramen is fresher and healthier than takeout yet just as satisfying. Miso paste provides deep savory notes that enhance store-bought vegetable broth. Swapping ramen noodles for the zucchini and adding fiber-packed broccoli and baby spinach ensures green vegetables in every bite. The jammy egg yolk melts into the broth, lending richness, and a splash of toasted sesame oil adds a delicious nuttiness.

> **Tip:** Miso is fermented soybean paste that comes in several varieties, any of which can be used for this soup. White miso is the mildest and sweetest. For an earthier version, try yellow miso, and for a deeper-flavored option, try red miso.

> **Tip:** To save time, look for packaged spiralized zucchini in your grocery store's produce section. If you're doing the work yourself, you can spiralize a couple days ahead. Keep your "zoodles" in an airtight container in the fridge.

4 large eggs
1 quart vegetable broth
5 ounces broccoli florets, cut into bite-size pieces (3 cups)
10 ounces (4 cups) spiralized zucchini
5 ounces baby spinach (5 packed cups)
1 tablespoon plus 2 teaspoons white miso paste
Kosher salt
1 tablespoon toasted sesame oil, plus more for garnish
2 cups mung bean sprouts, for garnish
Chili garlic sauce, for garnish

1. Lower the eggs into a large saucepan of gently boiling water and cook for 7 minutes, then transfer to a bowl of ice water.
2. Drain the cooking water from the saucepan, then add the broth and 2 cups of fresh water. Bring to a simmer over medium-high heat (do not boil). Add the broccoli and cook for 3 minutes, then add the zucchini and spinach. Continue cooking until the spinach is wilted and the zucchini is crisp-tender, 2 to 3 minutes more. Remove from the heat.
3. Ladle about ½ cup of the broth from the saucepan into a small bowl. Add the miso and ¼ teaspoon salt and whisk to combine. Return the

mixture to the soup, add the sesame oil, and stir to combine. Adjust the seasoning to taste. Cover to keep warm.

4. Remove the eggs from the ice bath; peel, then cut in half lengthwise. Ladle 2 cups of soup into each of four serving bowls. Top each portion with one egg and ½ cup sprouts. Drizzle with chili garlic sauce and more sesame oil to taste.

PER SERVING

ATKINS 20 • Net Carbs: 9 grams; Total Carbs: 15 grams; Fiber: 6 grams; Protein: 14 grams; Fat: 9 grams; Calories: 193; FV: 3

ATKINS 40 with ¼ cup shredded raw carrot and 1 tablespoon crushed peanuts on top per serving • Net Carbs: 10 grams; Total Carbs: 17 grams; Fiber: 7 grams; Protein: 16 grams; Fat: 13 grams; Calories: 253; FV: 4

ATKINS 100 with ¼ cup cooked rice noodles per serving • Net Carbs: 18 grams; Total Carbs: 25 grams; Fiber: 7 grams; Protein: 14 grams; Fat: 9 grams; Calories: 240; FV: 3

PROSCIUTTO CHICKEN WITH LOTS OF GREENS

SERVES 4 • TIME: Active—55 minutes Total—55 minutes

Traditional chicken saltimbocca relies on a coating of flour to achieve its crave-worthy crispness. In this version, we skip the flour and use prosciutto alone to add rich flavor and a crispy bite.

Tip: Chicken breasts vary in size and weight. Two larger breasts can be cut in half lengthwise to form four 6-ounce pieces, if needed. You can ask your butcher to cut and/or pound the breasts to save time.

··

Tip: *Swiss chard, along with kale, beet greens, spinach, or bok*
choy (alone or mixed) are all great options for the delicious,
quick-cooking greens.

··

5 garlic cloves

1 large lemon

1 tablespoon dried oregano

Kosher salt

¼ teaspoon freshly ground black pepper

2 tablespoons extra-virgin olive oil

4 (6-ounce) skinless, boneless chicken breast halves, gently pounded
  to ⅓-inch thickness

4 slices prosciutto (3 ounces)

2 bunches Swiss chard, (about 1¼ pounds), trimmed, stems very
  thinly sliced, leaves roughly chopped (about 10 cups)

1. Using a microplane or the smallest holes on a box grater, grate three
   of the garlic cloves and the zest of the lemon into a bowl. Stir in the
   oregano, 1 teaspoon salt, the pepper, and 1 tablespoon oil.
2. Slice the remaining 2 garlic cloves and juice the lemon. Set aside.
3. Rub the garlic–lemon zest mixture all over the chicken. Place one
   slice of prosciutto on each breast, pressing to help it adhere.
4. In a large skillet, heat the remaining 1 tablespoon of oil over medium-
   high heat. Add the chicken, prosciutto side down, in batches if necessary, and cook until the prosciutto side is crispy, 4 to 5 minutes. Turn
   the chicken and cook until the chicken is cooked through (an instant-
   read thermometer inserted into the thickest part will register 165°F),
   about 4 to 6 minutes more.
5. Transfer the chicken to four serving plates. Return the skillet to
   medium-high heat. Add the sliced garlic and the chard stems, cook

for 2 minutes, then add half of the leaves. Cook, stirring occasionally, until the chard begins to wilt, about 2 minutes. Add the remaining leaves, the lemon juice, and ¼ teaspoon salt. Cook until the chard is wilted, 2 to 3 minutes.

6. Transfer a quarter of the chard (about a heaping ½ cup) to each serving plate and serve.

PER SERVING

ATKINS 20 • Net Carbs: 3 grams; Total Carbs: 5 grams; Fiber: 2 grams; Protein: 46 grams; Fat: 13 grams; Calories: 330; FV: 2

ATKINS 40 with 2 tablespoons cooked polenta (prepared with water) per serving • Net Carbs: 9 grams; Total Carbs: 11 grams; Fiber: 2 grams; Protein: 47 grams; Fat: 13 grams; Calories: 358; FV: 2

ATKINS 100 with ⅓ cup cooked polenta (prepared with water) per serving • Net Carbs: 17 grams; Total Carbs: 20 grams; Fiber: 3 grams; Protein: 47 grams; Fat: 14 grams; Calories: 401; FV: 2

CRISPY CAJUN CHICKEN THIGHS WITH CELERY RANCH SALAD

SERVES 4 • TIME: Active—10 minutes Total—50 minutes

Here celery salad with a creamy DIY ranch dressing is the perfect cooling complement to Cajun-spiced chicken. Making our easy homemade dressing rather than using a store-bought version is a great way to cut down on carbs and added sodium and sugar. An added bonus: it's super delicious!

....

Tip: *Look for salt-free Cajun seasoning (a blend of paprika, cayenne, garlic powder, onion powder, and dried herbs), which allows you to control the sodium content of your dish.*

....

8 bone-in, skin-on chicken thighs (about 3 pounds)

2 tablespoons Cajun seasoning, preferably salt-free

Kosher salt

⅓ cup sour cream

2 tablespoons finely chopped fresh dill, plus more for garnish

1 tablespoon red wine vinegar

½ teaspoon garlic powder

Freshly ground black pepper

4 cups thinly, diagonally sliced celery, plus coarsely chopped leaves from the inner core

4 ounces blue cheese, crumbled (1 cup)

1. Preheat the oven to 425°F.
2. Pat the chicken dry with paper towels and rub with the Cajun seasoning and 1 teaspoon salt.
3. Place a wire rack over a rimmed baking sheet. Arrange the chicken on the rack, skin side up. Bake until crispy and cooked through (an instant-read thermometer inserted into the thickest part will register 165°F), 35 to 40 minutes.
4. Meanwhile, in a small bowl, stir together the sour cream, dill, vinegar, garlic powder, ½ teaspoon salt, and a pinch of pepper.
5. Place two chicken thighs and 1 cup of sliced celery on each of four serving plates. Dollop 1 heaping tablespoon of dressing on each plate of celery, then top each with the celery leaves, ¼ cup blue cheese, and dill to taste, and serve.

PER SERVING

ATKINS 20 • Net Carbs: 4 grams; Total Carbs: 5 grams; Fiber: 1 gram; Protein: 55 grams; Fat: 60 grams; Calories: 788; FV: 1

ATKINS 40 with ½ cup chopped raw carrots per serving added to the salad • Net Carbs: 8 grams; Total Carbs: 11 grams; Fiber: 3 grams; Protein: 55 grams; Fat: 60 grams; Calories: 814; FV: 6

ATKINS 100 *with 1 serving of Sweet Potato Fries per serving (recipe follows)*
• Net Carbs: 23 grams; Total Carbs: 28 grams; Fiber: 5 grams; Protein: 57
grams; Fat: 65 grams; Calories: 931; FV: 21

SWEET POTATO FRIES

SERVES 4

1 large sweet potato (about 1 pound), cut lengthwise into ¼- to
½-inch-wide sticks
1½ tablespoons olive oil
½ teaspoon kosher salt
¼ teaspoon freshly ground black pepper

Preheat the oven to 450°F. On a rimmed baking sheet, toss the sweet
potatoes with the oil, salt, and pepper, then arrange in a single layer.
Roast the sweet potatoes, flipping once halfway through, until golden
and tender, 25 to 30 minutes. Serve hot.

PER SERVING

Net Carbs: 19 grams; Total Carbs: 23 grams; Fiber: 4 grams; Protein: 2 grams;
Fat: 5 grams; Calories: 143; FV: 20

PAPRIKA PORK CHOPS WITH SAUERKRAUT
AND MUSTARD

SERVES 4 • TIME: *Active*—20 minutes *Total*—25 minutes

A blend of smoked paprika, garlic powder, and salt lends big flavor
to juicy pork chops, eliminating the need for a multihour marinade.
Combining melted butter with the savory pan juices makes for an easy
sauce. Sauerkraut pairs well with pork and lends immune-boosting

probiotics. And parsley, which is high in antioxidants and antibacterial compounds, makes for a pretty and tasty garnish. Round out this dish with a simple green salad.

··

Tip: *If you have a 12-inch skillet, you can cook all four chops at once; if you are using a smaller skillet, cook the chops in two batches.*

··

1½ teaspoons kosher salt

1½ teaspoons smoked paprika

¾ teaspoon garlic powder

4 (1½-inch-thick) bone-in pork chops (8 to 10 ounces each)

1 tablespoon neutral-flavored oil, such as canola

2 tablespoons unsalted butter

1⅓ cups sauerkraut

4 tablespoons whole grain or regular Dijon mustard

2 tablespoons finely chopped parsley

1. In a small bowl, combine the salt, paprika, and garlic powder. Pat the pork chops dry, then season them all over with the spice mixture.

2. In a large cast-iron or heavy stainless-steel skillet, heat the oil over medium-high heat until hot but not smoking. Add the pork chops, in two batches if necessary, and cook until the underside is golden, 1 to 2 minutes. Flip and cook 1 to 2 minutes more. Continue cooking, turning the chops every 1 to 2 minutes until the chops are deep golden and an instant-read thermometer inserted into the thickest part reads 145°F, 8 to 10 minutes total.

3. Transfer the pork chops to a cutting board; let rest for 5 minutes. Meanwhile, add the butter to the skillet and melt over medium heat; stir to combine with the pan drippings.

4. Place 1 pork chop, ⅓ cup sauerkraut, and 1 tablespoon mustard on each of four serving plates. Spoon ½ tablespoon of butter over each chop. Sprinkle each portion with ½ tablespoon parsley and serve.

PER SERVING

ATKINS 20 • Net Carbs: 2 grams; Total Carbs: 4 grams; Fiber: 2 grams;
Protein: 48 grams; Fat: 24 grams; Calories: 453; FV: 4

ATKINS 40 *with 1 serving of Cauliflower–Sour Cream Mash (recipe follows)* •
Net Carbs: 11 grams; Total Carbs: 16 grams; Fiber: 5 grams; Protein: 54
grams; Fat: 42 grams; Calories: 687; FV: 4

ATKINS 100 *with 1 serving of Sautéed Apples and Thyme (recipe follows)* •
Net Carbs: 11 grams; Total Carbs: 15 grams; Fiber: 4 grams; Protein:
49 grams; Fat: 28 grams; Calories: 531; FV: 4

CAULIFLOWER–SOUR CREAM MASH

SERVES 6

8 cups cauliflower florets
2 tablespoons sour cream
2 tablespoons heavy cream
1½ tablespoons unsalted butter
1 teaspoon kosher salt

1. In a large pot with a steamer basket, place the cauliflower florets into the basket and bring 1 cup of water to a boil over high heat. Cover tightly and cook until tender, 10 to 12 minutes. Drain.
2. In a food processor, puree the caulilflower, adding the florets in batches. Add the sour cream, heavy cream, butter, and salt and process until smooth and well combined. Reheat gently, if necessary, before serving.

PER SERVING

Net Carbs: 4 grams; Total Carbs: 7 grams; Fiber: 3 grams; Protein: 3 grams;
Fat: 4 grams; Calories: 85; FV: 4

SAUTÉED APPLES AND THYME

SERVES 4

2 Gala or Fuji apples, cut into ¼-inch cubes (2 cups total)
1½ tablespoons unsalted butter
Kosher salt
Freshly ground black pepper
Dried thyme

In a medium skillet over medium-high heat, sauté the apples in the butter with a pinch each of salt, pepper, and thyme until the apple is warm and crisp-tender, 5 to 7 minutes. Remove from the heat. Serve a heaping ½ cup of warm apples with each pork chop.

PER SERVING

Net Carbs: 9 grams; Total Carbs: 11 grams; Fiber: 2 grams; Protein: 1 gram; Fat: 4 grams; Calories: 78; FV: 0

"NACHOS" STUFFED CHICKEN BREAST

SERVES 4 • TIME: *Active*—30 minutes *Total*—50 minutes

If a tray of cheesy nachos is your go-to pub snack, this winning chicken dinner is for you. Here, chicken breasts are stuffed with sour cream, shredded cheese, and fresh herbs and baked until golden. A chopped tomato and fresh cilantro topping rounds out the full "nacho" effect. As the chicken bakes, you'll whip up a zesty salad. If your market sells "power greens" or "superfood greens" (often a tasty mix of nutrient-dense baby greens, such as spinach, chard, and kale), give them a try.

....

Tip: *If you prefer a mild dish, substitute cheddar for the Pepper Jack cheese. If you want an extra-spicy dish, add a tablespoon of your favorite Mexican hot sauce to the filling before stuffing the chicken breasts.*

....

4 ounces shredded Pepper Jack cheese (1 cup)

⅓ cup sour cream

1 scallion, thinly sliced

2 tablespoons finely chopped cilantro, plus more for garnish

Kosher salt

4 boneless, skinless chicken breasts (about 2 pounds total)

2 teaspoons chili powder

Nonstick cooking spray

1 medium tomato, finely chopped (⅔ cup)

For the greens and dressing

¼ cup fresh lime juice (from 2 large limes)

3 tablespoons extra-virgin olive oil

½ teaspoon granulated erythritol

Kosher salt

Freshly ground black pepper

5 packed cups baby greens

1. Preheat the oven to 400°F.

2. In a small bowl, combine the cheese, sour cream, scallion, cilantro, and ½ teaspoon salt.

3. Insert a small sharp knife into the thickest part of each chicken breast and push it three-quarters of the way down to the thin end, being careful not to pierce the outside of the breast. Move the knife from side to side to form a wide pocket with a narrow opening. Stuff each

breast with a quarter of the cheese mixture (about ¼ cup). Secure with toothpicks. Season the chicken with the chili powder and 1 teaspoon salt.

4. Lightly coat a large ovenproof skillet with cooking spray and heat over medium-high heat until hot but not smoking. Place the chicken breasts into the skillet and cook until golden, about 2 minutes per side. Transfer the skillet to the oven and roast until an instant-read thermometer inserted into the thickest part of the breast reads 165°F, 18 to 20 minutes.

5. Meanwhile, prepare the dressing: In a small bowl, whisk the lime juice, oil, erythritol, and a generous pinch each of salt and pepper together until combined.

6. Remove the chicken from the oven. Remove and discard the tooth-picks, then arrange the chicken on four serving plates. Mound 1¼ cups greens alongside each chicken breast, then drizzle the greens with about 1½ tablespoons of dressing per serving. Top each portion with 2 heaping tablespoons of chopped tomato and cilantro to taste and serve.

PER SERVING

ATKINS 20 • Net Carbs: 5 grams; Total Carbs: 7 grams; Fiber: 2 grams;
  Protein: 59 grams; Fat: 28 grams; Calories: 520; FV: 1

ATKINS 40 *with 2 tablespoons canned refried black beans per*
  serving • Net Carbs: 9 grams; Total Carbs: 12 grams; Fiber: 3 grams;
  Protein: 60 grams; Fat: 28 grams; Calories: 545; FV: 1

ATKINS 100 *with ½ cup canned refried black beans per serving* • Net Carbs:
  18 grams; Total Carbs: 26 grams; Fiber: 8 grams; Protein: 65 grams;
  Fat: 29 grams; Calories: 620; FV: 1

VIETNAMESE GLAZED CHICKEN THIGHS WITH CABBAGE SALAD

SERVES 4 • TIME: *Active*—20 minutes *Total*—55 minutes

In this Vietnamese-inspired chicken dinner, an umami-packed sauce made with soy sauce, fish sauce, rice vinegar, and chili-garlic paste plays double duty as a marinade for the chicken and a dressing for the salad. If you're meal prepping for the week, you can marinate the chicken in the fridge overnight. Otherwise, let the chicken marinate at least 30 minutes before cooking to infuse it with as much flavor as possible. Chinese cabbage, also called Napa cabbage, is sweeter and softer than green cabbage, making it the perfect choice for a raw, crunchy salad. It's also packed with vitamins C and K and fiber. Leftover leaves can be used for stuffed cabbage or for making a nutrient-dense dumpling filling.

·····························

Tip: *For a less intense heat, remove the seeds and ribs from the serrano pepper.*

·····························

Tip: *The sweetness of erythritol gives this dish its characteristic funky-sweet tang, but you can leave it out and have an equally delicious dish.*

·····························

⅓ cup rice wine vinegar

3 tablespoons soy sauce

3 tablespoons fish sauce

1 tablespoon chili-garlic paste (such as sambal oelek)

1 tablespoon granulated erythritol

2 pounds boneless, skinless chicken thighs

2 tablespoons olive oil

8 cups shredded Chinese cabbage (from a 1-pound head)

2 scallions, thinly sliced

¼ cup chopped fresh mint leaves, plus more for serving
¼ cup chopped fresh cilantro leaves, plus more for serving
1 large serrano or jalapeño pepper, thinly sliced (about ¼ cup)

1. In a bowl, whisk together the vinegar, soy sauce, fish sauce, chili-garlic paste, and erythritol. In a second bowl, add the chicken and cover with half of the vinegar mixture (about ⅓ cup). Cover and refrigerate the remaining vinegar mixture for the salad dressing.
2. Marinate the chicken pieces for 30 minutes at room temperature or up to 24 hours covered and refrigerated. (If you marinate the chicken in the refrigerator, allow it to come to room temperature for 30 minutes before cooking.)
3. Set an oven rack 5 to 6 inches from the heat source. Preheat the broiler to high.
4. Remove the chicken pieces from the marinade and place them on a rimmed baking sheet. Drizzle with 1 tablespoon of oil. Broil 6 to 8 minutes per side or until the chicken is lightly golden and cooked through (an instant-read thermometer inserted into the thickest part will register 165°F).
5. Meanwhile, add 1 tablespoon of water and 1 tablespoon of oil to the reserved marinade and whisk to combine; this is the dressing. In a large bowl, toss together the cabbage, scallions, mint, cilantro, serrano pepper, and dressing. Arrange 2 heaping cups of salad on each of four serving plates.
6. Allow the chicken to rest for 5 minutes, then slice. Place about a quarter of the chicken on top of each salad. Top with additional herbs, if desired, and serve.

PER SERVING

ATKINS 20 • Net Carbs: 7 grams; Total Carbs: 9 grams; Fiber: 2 grams; Protein: 49 grams; Fat: 15 grams; Calories: 360; FV: 1

ATKINS 40 *with 1½ tablespoons chopped salted peanuts per serving* • Net
  Carbs: 8 grams; Total Carbs: 11 grams; Fiber: 3 grams; Protein: 53 grams;
  Fat: 22 grams; Calories: 440; FV: 1

ATKINS 100 *with ½ sliced grapefruit added to the salad per serving* • Net
  Carbs: 18 grams; Total Carbs: 21 grams; Fiber: 3 grams; Protein: 50 grams;
  Fat: 15 grams; Calories: 406; FV: 1

SEARED HANGER STEAK WITH HARISSA BUTTER AND SPINACH

SERVES 4 • TIME: *Active—*25 minutes *Total—*25 minutes

The secret ingredient in this gorgeous steak dinner is a simple flavored butter made with zippy jarred harissa (a North African chili paste) and lemon zest. When it melts over the warm steak, it's heaven. A healthy sauté of spinach makes the perfect easy side and recalls the classic steak house pairing.

....

Tip: *Look for harissa in the international section of gourmet shops and larger grocery stores, or buy it online.*

....

Tip: *The best way to eliminate guesswork regarding steak doneness is to use an instant-read thermometer. Go for 130°F for medium rare; 135°F to 140°F for medium; and 145°F to 150°F for medium well done.*

....

2 (1-pound) hanger steaks at room temperature
Kosher salt
Freshly ground black pepper
2½ tablespoons unsalted butter at room temperature
1½ teaspoons harissa

½ teaspoon grated lemon zest

2 tablespoons extra-virgin olive oil

8 cups packed chopped spinach (12 ounces)

2 tablespoons fresh lemon juice

1. Season the steaks generously with salt and pepper.
2. In a small bowl, stir together the butter, harissa, lemon zest, and ⅛ teaspoon salt until well combined.
3. Heat a large skillet, preferably cast iron, over medium-high heat until hot, 2 to 3 minutes. Add 1 tablespoon of oil, then the steaks. Cook until golden on the underside, about 5 minutes, then flip and cook until an instant-read thermometer inserted into the thickest part registers 135°F for medium, 3 to 5 minutes more depending on the thickness. Transfer the steaks to a cutting board. Top with the butter and let rest for 5 to 10 minutes.
4. Meanwhile, in the same skillet, heat 1 tablespoon of oil over medium heat. Add half of the spinach and cook until wilted, 1 to 2 minutes, then add the remaining spinach and the lemon juice. Continue cooking, stirring, until the spinach is wilted, 1 to 2 minutes more. Adjust the seasoning to taste.
5. Place a heaping ¼ cup spinach on each of four serving plates. Slice the steak, transfer about ½ pound to each plate, and serve.

PER SERVING

ATKINS 20 • Net Carbs: 3 grams; Total Carbs: 4 grams; Fiber: 1 gram; Protein: 66 grams; Fat: 34 grams; Calories: 583; FV: 1

ATKINS 40 *with ¼ cup rinsed and drained canned cannellini beans per serving* • Net Carbs: 9 grams; Total Carbs: 15 grams; Fiber: 6 grams; Protein: 70 grams; Fat: 34 grams; Calories: 643; FV: 1

ATKINS 100 *with ½ cup rinsed and drained canned cannellini beans per serving* • Net Carbs: 14 grams; Total Carbs: 25 grams; Fiber: 11 grams; Protein: 74 grams; Fat: 34 grams; Calories: 703; FV: 1

LEMON BAKED COD WITH BRAISED CAULIFLOWER AND GREENS

SERVES 4 • TIME: *Active—*40 minutes *Total—*40 minutes

Spooning a lemony mayonnaise over cod before baking the fish lends delicious flavor and renders it juicy and moist. While the fish bakes, a flavorful side dish of skillet-braised cauliflower and Swiss chard comes together in minutes. These vegetables make a delicious combination and together offer a good dose of vitamins K and C and folate.

....

Tip: If cod is not available, substitute mahi mahi, sea bass, hake, or haddock.

....

Tip: If Swiss chard is not available or you want a change of pace, try spinach, kale, or escarole.

....

Nonstick cooking spray
1 large lemon
⅓ cup mayonnaise
4 (6-ounce) cod fillets, about 1 inch thick
Kosher salt
Freshly ground black pepper
1 tablespoon extra-virgin olive oil
4 cups 1-inch cauliflower florets (from a 1½-pound head)
½ cup low-sodium chicken broth
1½ teaspoons finely chopped flat anchovy fillet
2 bunches Swiss chard (about 1½ pounds), leaves and tender stems coarsely chopped

1. Set an oven rack in the middle position. Preheat the oven to 400°F. Lightly coat a 9-by-12-inch baking dish with nonstick cooking spray.

2. Grate enough zest from the lemon to yield 1 teaspoon. Cut off a small piece of the lemon from one end and squeeze to yield 1 teaspoon of juice. In a small bowl, stir together the mayonnaise, lemon zest, and lemon juice. Cut the remaining lemon into wedges.

3. Season the cod with ½ teaspoon salt and ¼ teaspoon pepper. Spread the mayonnaise mixture over the tops and sides of the fish and arrange in the prepared baking dish. Add the lemon wedges. Bake until the cod is opaque and cooked through and an instant-read thermometer inserted into the thickest part registers 145°F, 15 to 20 minutes depending on the thickness.

4. Meanwhile, in a large skillet, heat the oil over medium-high heat. Add the cauliflower and cook, stirring occasionally, until it begins to turn golden, about 6 minutes. Add the broth, anchovy, and a generous pinch of salt. Cover, reduce the heat to medium, and cook until the cauliflower is crisp-tender, about 3 minutes.

5. Uncover the skillet and add the chard, in batches if necessary, and 1 to 2 tablespoons of water if the skillet is dry. Cook uncovered until the chard is wilted, 3 to 4 minutes. Season the vegetables to taste with salt and pepper.

6. Place one fillet of fish and 1¼ cups of vegetables on each of four plates. Squeeze the baked lemon pieces over the top.

PER SERVING

ATKINS 20 • Net Carbs: 9 grams; Total Carbs: 15 grams; Fiber: 6 grams; Protein: 33 grams; Fat: 17 grams; Calories: 334; FV: 7

ATKINS 40 *with ¼ cup mashed cooked turnips per serving* • Net Carbs: 11 grams; Total Carbs: 18 grams; Fiber: 7 grams; Protein: 33 grams; Fat: 17 grams; Calories: 347; FV: 9

ATKINS 100 *with ⅓ cup cooked quinoa (cooked in water) per serving* • Net Carbs: 19 grams; Total Carbs: 27 grams; Fiber: 8 grams; Protein: 35 grams; Fat: 18 grams; Calories: 403; FV: 7

QUICK SEAFOOD STEW WITH BASIL PISTOU

SERVES 4 • TIME: *Active*—15 minutes *Total*—40 minutes

French basil pistou is Italian pesto's lesser-known cousin—a similar sauce but classically made without nuts. Here it's hand chopped and spooned over a hearty stew of shrimp, cod, and escarole, providing a heady, herbal aroma and flavor.

4 tablespoons extra-virgin olive oil
½ cup finely chopped celery
2 tablespoons finely chopped yellow onion
2 large garlic cloves, grated
Kosher salt
1 quart low-sodium vegetable stock
1 cup bottled clam juice
½ cup drained canned diced tomatoes or peeled chopped fresh
   tomato
2 bay leaves
1 cup packed fresh basil leaves, finely chopped
½ teaspoon grated lemon zest
1 pound large shrimp, peeled and deveined
12 ounces cod, cut into 1½-inch cubes
1½ cups coarsely chopped escarole
1 tablespoon unsalted butter
1 lemon, quartered, for garnish

1. In a heavy, wide pot, heat 1 tablespoon of oil over medium heat. Add the celery and onion and cook, stirring frequently, until softened, 2 to 3 minutes. Add three-quarters of the garlic and a pinch of salt. Continue to cook, stirring, for 30 seconds, then add the vegetable

stock, clam juice, tomatoes, bay leaves, and ¾ teaspoon salt. Bring to a boil over high heat, then reduce to a simmer and cook until flavorful and slightly reduced, about 15 minutes.

2. Meanwhile, stir together the basil, the lemon zest, 3 tablespoons olive oil, the remaining garlic, and ¼ teaspoon salt (this is the pistou).

3. Add the shrimp and cod to the pot with the tomato liquid, cover, and cook over medium heat for 2 minutes. Remove the cover and stir in the escarole and butter. Cook until the fish is opaque and cooked through and the escarole is wilted, 1 to 2 minutes. Remove and discard the bay leaves.

4. Remove the soup from the heat and ladle 2 cups into each of four serving bowls. Top each bowl with 1 tablespoon of pistou. Squeeze the lemon wedges over the top and serve.

PER SERVING

ATKINS 20 • Net Carbs: 9 grams; Total Carbs: 12 grams; Fiber: 3 grams; Protein: 30 grams; Fat: 18 grams; Calories: 330; FV: 2

ATKINS 40 *with 1 tablespoon sliced almonds per serving* • Net Carbs: 11 grams; Total Carbs: 13 grams; Fiber: 4 grams; Protein: 31 grams; Fat: 21 grams; Calories: 363; FV: 2

ATKINS 100 *with ¼ small toasted Au Bon Pain multigrain baguette per serving* • Net Carbs: 17 grams; Total Carbs: 22 grams; Fiber: 5 grams; Protein: 33 grams; Fat: 22 grams; Calories: 408; FV: 2

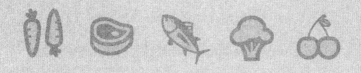

RECIPES

ATKINS 20

ATKINS 40

ATKINS 100

CHAPTER 11

SNACKS

Savory and Sweet, Cheesy and Crunchy Bites

WHETHER YOU NEED a quick low-carb bite to keep your hunger under control, calm a craving, or you want a tasty appetizer before your main meal, these recipes will give you an appealing array of delectable finger food.

The recipes in this chapter are categorized under Atkins 20, Atkins 40, and Atkins 100.

CHEESY CAULIFLOWER BITES

SERVES 6 • TIME: *Active*—40 minutes *Total*—55 minutes

An excellent source of vitamin C and a good source of folate and vitamin B_6, cauliflower pairs well with cheese. Here the duo is made into satisfying bites that make a great game-day snack. If you don't have a mini muffin tin, form the mixture into tablespoon-size patties and bake them on a parchment paper–lined baking sheet.

Nonstick cooking spray

Kosher salt

4 cups bite-size cauliflower florets (12 ounces) or 12 ounces frozen
　　cauliflower rice (not thawed)

4 ounces shredded low-moisture mozzarella cheese (1 cup)

½ cup plus 2 tablespoons freshly grated Parmesan cheese

1 large egg, lightly beaten

2 tablespoons chopped chives or scallions

¼ teaspoon garlic powder

¼ teaspoon red pepper flakes

Freshly ground black pepper

1. Preheat the oven to 400°F. Lightly coat a 24-cup mini muffin tin with nonstick cooking spray.

2. If using cauliflower florets, bring a large pot of salted water to a boil. Add the cauliflower and cook until very tender, 3 to 4 minutes, then drain in a colander. Transfer to a plate and let cool completely. Pat dry with paper towels. In the bowl of a food processor, pulse the cauliflower until it resembles ricelike granules. Transfer to a clean dishcloth and wring out as much water as possible (you will have 1 cup cooked riced cauliflower).

3. If using frozen cauliflower rice, cook according to the package instructions. Transfer to a clean dishcloth and wring out as much water as possible (you will have 1 cup cooked riced cauliflower).

4. In a large bowl, stir together the cooked cauliflower, mozzarella, ½ cup Parmesan, egg, chives or scallion, garlic powder, red pepper flakes, ¼ teaspoon salt, and a generous pinch of pepper.

5. Divide the mixture among the muffin cups (about 1 tablespoon in each), and sprinkle with 2 tablespoons of Parmesan. Bake until golden, 15 to 17 minutes.

6. Take the tin from the oven. Turn out the cauliflower bites and serve four warm bites per person.

PER SERVING

ATKINS 20 • Net Carbs: 5 grams; Total Carbs: 6 grams; Fiber: 1 gram;
Protein: 9 grams; Fat: 9 grams; Calories: 135; FV: 2

ZUCCHINI FRITTERS WITH SUN-DRIED TOMATO PESTO

SERVES 4 • TIME: *Active*—50 minutes *Total*—50 minutes
Makes 8 fritters

These crispy warm fritters combine zucchini with the classic Italian trio of tomato, basil, and mozzarella cheese to create a veggie-packed, satisfying snack that's fun to make and share.

....

Tip: Low-moisture mozzarella cheese is a denser, drier version of mozzarella sold in blocks or preshredded in bags. Don't confuse it with fresh mozzarella, which is sold in balls.

....

Tip: To keep the fritters warm between batches, arrange on a cooling rack set inside a rimmed baking sheet and place in a 225°F oven.

....

For the fritters
  2 medium zucchini (1 pound total), grated on the large
     holes of a box grater
  Kosher salt
  2 ounces shredded low-moisture mozzarella cheese (½ cup)
  ½ cup freshly grated Parmesan cheese (1.6 ounces)
  ¼ cup finely-chopped fresh basil leaves
  1 large egg, lightly beaten
  ¼ teaspoon garlic powder
  Freshly ground black pepper
  2 tablespoons neutral-flavored oil, such as canola

For the pesto

   2½ tablespoons sun-dried tomatoes packed in oil (1¼ ounces),
      drained and thinly sliced
   2 tablespoons packed fresh basil leaves (⅛ ounce), thinly sliced
   ½ garlic clove, thinly sliced
   1½ tablespoons freshly grated Parmesan cheese
   Kosher salt
   2 tablespoons extra-virgin olive oil

1. Prepare the pesto: On a cutting board, mound the sun-dried tomatoes, basil, and garlic. Finely chop and scrape together to form a paste.
   Transfer the paste to a bowl. Stir in the Parmesan and ⅛ teaspoon salt
   to combine, then stir in the olive oil in 2 additions, stirring well in
   between to combine. Set aside.

2. Prepare the fritters: In a colander set in the sink or over a bowl, add
   the grated zucchini and toss with ¼ teaspoon of salt, then let stand
   10 to 15 minutes to drain. (You can do this step before you make the
   pesto, if you prefer.)

3. Firmly press the zucchini with the back of a large spoon to release
   as much liquid as possible, then wrap it in a clean kitchen towel and
   wring out the remaining liquid (you will have about 1 cup packed
   zucchini). Discard the liquid.

4. In a dry bowl, add the zucchini, mozzarella, Parmesan, basil, egg, garlic powder, ¼ teaspoon salt, and a generous pinch of pepper, and stir
   to combine.

5. In a large nonstick skillet, heat 1 tablespoon of canola oil over
   medium-high heat until shimmering. Add the zucchini batter in ¼
   cup portions, about four at a time, pressing each to slightly flatten
   it, and cook until golden and crisp on the bottom, 2 to 3 minutes.
   (Reduce the heat if the fritters brown too quickly.) Carefully flip the
   fritters and continue cooking until the second side is golden, 2 to
   3 minutes more. Transfer the fritters to a paper towel–lined plate,

season with salt to taste, and repeat with the remaining oil and fritters.

6. Stir the pesto together to combine (since this is a hand-chopped pesto, it isn't as smooth as a blender version and tends to separate). Serve 2 warm fritters with 1 tablespoon of pesto for each serving.

PER SERVING

ATKINS 20 • Net Carbs: 4 grams; Total Carbs: 6 grams; Fiber: 1 gram; Protein: 8 grams; Fat: 22 grams; Calories: 246; FV: 2

GREEN GODDESS GUACAMOLE WITH CRUNCHY VEGGIES

SERVES 4 • TIME: *Active*—25 minutes *Total*—30 minutes

The only thing better than classic restaurant-style guacamole? This homemade version packed with creamy avocados and fresh herbs. A great source of folate, fiber, and vitamin B_6, avocados make a satisfying midday nosh. An assortment of crisp veggies—nature's tortilla chips!—are used for dipping.

. . . .

Tip: For a milder guacamole, use less of the pepper or omit it altogether. For a spicier version, double up!

. . . .

Kosher salt

3 ounces sugar snap peas (about 1 cup), strings removed

2 large avocados (1 pound total)

3 tablespoons chopped fresh chives or scallion

1 tablespoon grated lemon zest

3 tablespoons fresh lime juice (from 2 limes)

1 tablespoon finely chopped seeded jalapeño pepper

2 teaspoons finely chopped fresh cilantro

1 small garlic clove, minced

2 endives, leaves separated (1 cup)

4 Persian or 1½ English cucumbers, cut into spears

1. Bring a large pot of salted water to a boil. Fill a large bowl with ice water.
2. Add the peas to the boiling water and cook until bright green, about 1 minute. Drain and transfer to the ice water. Let stand 5 minutes, then drain and pat dry.
3. Halve and pit the avocados and scoop the flesh into a bowl. Mash the avocados with a fork and stir in the chives or scallion, lemon zest, lime juice, jalapeño, cilantro, garlic, and ¾ teaspoon salt.
4. Arrange the peas, endive, and cucumbers on a platter. Serve with the guacamole, about ¼ cup per person.

PER SERVING

ATKINS 20 • Net Carbs: 4 grams; Total Carbs: 12 grams; Fiber: 8 grams; Protein: 4 grams; Fat: 11 grams; Calories: 146; FV: 4

DUKKAH "DEVILED" EGGS

SERVES 6 • TIME: *Active—*20 minutes *Total—*30 minutes

This "lazy" version of classic deviled eggs is quicker than the classic but just as good. Instead of mashing the boiled yolks with mayonnaise, you simply spoon the mayo on top, then sprinkle with a toasty (and tasty!) homemade mix of spiced heart-healthy nuts and iron-rich seeds known as dukkah. Dukkah keeps well and can be made ahead. You can easily customize the servings for this snack, making as few as one serving at a time or doubling or tripling the recipe if you're serving a crowd.

....
Tip: Dukkah, an Egyptian blend of toasted nuts, seeds, and spices, keeps, covered and at cool room temperature, up to two weeks.
....

6 large eggs
2 walnut halves (⅛ ounce)
3 raw unsalted almonds (⅛ ounce)
½ teaspoon sesame seeds
⅛ teaspoon ground coriander
⅛ teaspoon ground cumin
Kosher salt
Freshly ground black pepper
¼ cup mayonnaise

1. Lower the eggs into a large saucepan of gently boiling water and cook for 8 minutes, then transfer to a bowl of ice water. Let stand for 5 minutes.
2. Meanwhile, in a small skillet over medium heat, toast the walnuts and almonds, stirring frequently, until fragrant and lightly golden, 3 to 4 minutes. Add the sesame seeds and cook, stirring occasionally, until toasted, 1 to 2 minutes more. Take the skillet from the heat.
3. On a cutting board, chop the nut mixture very finely, then transfer to a small bowl. Add the coriander, the cumin, and a very small pinch each of salt and pepper. Stir to combine. This is the dukkah.
4. Peel and cut the eggs in half lengthwise. Top each egg half with 1 teaspoon of the mayonnaise and ¼ teaspoon of the dukkah. Two egg halves with all the fixings make one serving.

PER SERVING

ATKINS 40 • Net Carbs: 1 gram; Total Carbs: 1 gram; Fiber: 0 grams; Protein: 6 grams; Fat: 12 grams; Calories: 141; FV: 0

MEZZE PLATE WITH FALAFEL-SPICED YOGURT DIP

SERVES 4 · TIME: *Active*—20 minutes *Total*—20 minutes

Here the flavors of falafel (a popular Middle Eastern chickpea patty) spice up a creamy, protein-powered yogurt dip that's delicious with crunchy vegetables and olive bar favorites such as marinated artichokes and makes a quick, beautiful, crave-worthy spread.

....
Tip: Look for mixed Greek olives in jars or at the olive bar
of larger grocery stores, where you can mix and match olive
varieties as you like.
....

2 ounces feta cheese, cubed (½ cup)
½ teaspoon dried oregano
2 tablespoons plus ½ teaspoon olive oil
½ cup plain full-fat Greek yogurt
1 tablespoon fresh lemon juice
1 small garlic clove, grated (½ teaspoon)
⅛ teaspoon ground cumin
⅛ teaspoon ground coriander
Kosher salt
2 Persian cucumbers or 1 English cucumber (6 ounces), cut into spears
4 small radishes, preferably with green tops, halved or quartered
  if large
⅓ cup jarred marinated artichoke hearts (2 ounces)
⅓ cup mixed olives (2 ounces)

1. In a small bowl, combine the feta, oregano, and 2 tablespoons of oil. Set aside to marinate at least 10 minutes at room temperature or refrigerated overnight.

2. Meanwhile, in a small bowl, stir together the yogurt, lemon juice, garlic, cumin, coriander, ¼ teaspoon salt, and ½ teaspoon oil. Adjust the salt to taste.

3. Place the bowl of yogurt on a serving platter. Arrange the cucumbers, radishes, artichoke hearts, and olives around the bowl. Using a slotted spoon, transfer the feta to the platter, then drizzle the feta oil over the dip and vegetables. Alternatively, a quarter of the vegetables, 2 heaping tablespoons of dip, and about 1 tablespoon of feta can be presented as one serving.

PER SERVING

ATKINS 40 • Net Carbs: 5 grams; Total Carbs: 6 grams; Fiber: 1 gram; Protein: 6 grams; Fat: 14 grams; Calories: 168; FV: 2

WEDGE SALAD CUPS

SERVES 4 • TIME: Active—30 minutes Total—40 minutes

This fun-to-eat snack version of a steak house wedge salad is filled with juicy tomatoes; fiber-rich asparagus; smoky, crisp bacon; crunchy cucumbers; and a creamy blue cheese dressing made with protein-packed Greek yogurt. To tote these to work or school or to a picnic or potluck, pack the dressing separately and spoon it into the cups just before serving.

Tip: To easily separate the iceberg lettuce leaves to make the cups, use a knife to carefully remove the core from the head, then hold the head, core face up, under cool running water, gently loosening and pulling apart the leaves.

Tip: Check the ingredients in your bacon to make sure it's sugar free.

....

*Tip: Cherry tomatoes tend to be good quality year round.
During the summer tomato season, feel free to substitute the
best varieties of regular tomatoes that you can find. Cut them
into cubes or small wedges, as you like.*

....

*Tip: Peel and discard the waxy skins from conventional
cucumbers, or use the Persian or English variety (both have
tender, unwaxed skins) and leave the skins on.*

....

For the lettuce cup filling

  10 medium stalks asparagus, trimmed and cut into 1-inch lengths
    (1 cup)
  5 ounces no-sugar-added bacon (5 to 8 strips, depending on thickness)
  8 medium iceberg lettuce leaves (see tip above)
  1 cup halved cherry tomatoes (6 ounces)
  1 cup cubed cucumber
  2 tablespoons chopped chives or scallions, for garnish

For the dressing

  ¼ cup mayonnaise
  ¼ cup full-fat Greek yogurt or sour cream
  1 tablespoon fresh lemon juice
  ¼ teaspoon garlic powder
  Kosher salt
  Freshly ground black pepper
  2 ounces crumbled blue cheese (½ cup)

1. Prepare the filling: In a large pot filled with about 1 inch of water, set a
   steamer basket. Cover the pot and bring the water to a boil over high
   heat. Place the asparagus in the steamer basket and steam, covered,
   until crisp-tender, 2 to 3 minutes for thin spears and 4 to 5 minutes

for thick ones. Remove the pot from the heat. Transfer the asparagus to a plate and let cool.

2. Meanwhile, in a large cast-iron skillet, arrange the bacon in a single layer and cook over medium heat, turning the bacon occasionally, until crispy, 10 to 12 minutes. Take the skillet from the heat and transfer the bacon to a paper towel–lined plate. Let cool, then crumble into pieces.

3. Prepare the dressing: In a small bowl, stir together the mayonnaise, yogurt or sour cream, lemon juice, garlic powder, ¼ teaspoon salt, and several grinds of pepper until combined. Stir in the blue cheese. Adjust the salt to taste.

4. Assemble the cups: Fill each lettuce cup with ⅛ cup tomatoes, 1 tablespoon asparagus, 1 heaping tablespoon bacon, and ⅛ cup cucumber. Top with 1 heaping tablespoon of dressing, a heaping ½ teaspoon chives or scallions, and pepper to taste. Plate two lettuce cups for each serving.

PER SERVING

ATKINS 40 • Net Carbs: 4 grams; Total Carbs: 6 grams; Fiber: 2 grams; Protein: 10 grams; Fat: 35 grams; Calories: 375; FV: 3

CHILI-SPICED PAPAYA

SERVES 6 • TIME: *Active*—15 minutes *Total*—15 minutes

Three simple ingredients are all it takes to bring juicy, antioxidant-rich papaya wedges to life: lime, ancho chili powder, and flaky sea salt. Zest the lime first, then cut it in half and squeeze the tangy juice over the papaya. Ancho chili powder provides a smokier flavor and milder heat than basic chili powder, but you can use any chili powder you like. A ripe papaya will be mostly yellow-orange in color and will give slightly when pressed.

····························

Tip: *To speed up the ripening process, place a papaya in a brown paper bag with a banana. The seeds of papayas are edible. Eat them raw or freeze or dry them, if desired, to add crunch to salads or other dishes.*

····························

½ medium papaya, peeled, seeded, and cut into 12 ½-inch wedges
   (12 ounces)

1 teaspoon lime zest

1 tablespoon fresh lime juice

½ teaspoon ancho or regular chili powder

¼ teaspoon flaky sea salt, such as Maldon

Arrange the papaya wedges on a platter. Sprinkle with lime zest, then top with the lime juice, chili powder, and sea salt. Plate two wedges for each serving.

PER SERVING

ATKINS 100 • Net Carbs: 9 grams; Total Carbs: 11 grams; Fiber: 2 grams;
   Protein: .5 gram; Fat: .2 gram; Calories: 45; FV: 0

BAKED BRIE WITH WARM GRAPES AND THYME

SERVES 6 • TIME: *Active*—20 minutes *Total*—40 minutes

A wheel of oozy, warm cheese is a creamy, comforting crowd pleaser, especially when paired with crisp homemade crostini. Balsamic vinegar–glazed grapes are easy to make and add a pop of juicy natural sweetness. This winner is a great one to share with friends at a book club get-together or on game or movie night.

····························

Tip: *Look for nutrient-dense Ezekiel bread in the freezer aisle of large grocery stores. Let it thaw completely in the fridge before toasting.*

····························

....
Tip: *Heat the Brie just long enough to warm it through. If it bakes for too long, serve it from a shallow bowl with a spoon for scooping; it won't hold its shape on a cheese board, but it will still be delicious!*
....

1 (6½-ounce) wheel Brie cheese

4 slices Ezekiel sprouted grain bread (5.5 ounces), thawed if frozen

3 tablespoons olive oil, divided

Kosher salt

Freshly ground black pepper

½ cup seedless red grapes, washed and dried (2½ ounces)

1½ teaspoons balsamic vinegar

¾ teaspoon finely chopped fresh thyme leaves

1. Set oven racks in the upper and lower third positions. Preheat the oven to 350°F. Place the Brie on a parchment-lined baking sheet and set aside.

2. Cut the bread slices into 6 pieces each, similar in size to a small toast point or crostini, brush both sides of the pieces with 2½ tablespoons of oil, and season with a pinch each of salt and pepper. Arrange in a single layer on a second baking sheet.

3. Bake the bread on the lower oven rack until the undersides are golden and crisp, 12 to 15 minutes. Flip the bread pieces, rotate the baking sheet, return it to the lower rack, and continue baking until the bread is golden and crisp, 5 to 7 minutes more.

4. Meanwhile, place the Brie on the top rack and bake until warmed through but not oozing, 7 to 10 minutes.

5. While the bread and Brie are baking heat ½ tablespoon of oil, in a large skillet, over medium-high heat until hot but not smoking. Add the grapes and cook, tossing, until the skins begin to split, 3 to 4 minutes. Reduce the heat to medium low and carefully add the vinegar (it will bubble), thyme, and a pinch each of salt and pepper. Cook until the liquid is reduced and the grapes are warm, 3 to 5 minutes.

6. Remove the bread and cheese from the oven and arrange on a platter. Spoon the grapes along with any syrup from the pan over the cheese. Alternatively, plate four "crostini" with a sixth of the cheese wheel topped with grapes for each serving. Serve immediately.

PER SERVING

ATKINS 100 • Net Carbs: 11 grams; Total Carbs: 13 grams; Fiber: 2 grams; Protein: 9 grams; Fat: 16 grams; Calories: 228; FV: 0

PEACH CAPRESE SKEWERS

SERVES 4 • TIME: *Active*—25 minutes *Total*—25 minutes

Here we're giving classic caprese skewers an upgrade by adding sliced fresh peach, prosciutto, and a drizzle of herby pesto. The quickest way to make these is to prep all the ingredients first, then set up an assembly line to thread the ingredients onto skewers. (To make it even quicker, share the fun with a friend or a willing kid or two!) If you take these to a potluck or backyard barbecue, pack the pesto separately and do the drizzling just before serving.

....

Tip: *Look for small fresh mozzarella balls, called bocconcini, in the cheese department at large grocery stores and at cheese shops.*

....

Tip: *If peaches are not in season, frozen can be used. Thaw them before skewering.*

....

Tip: *Persian cucumbers are small cukes that have a crisp bite and pleasingly tender skins. If they're not available, any good cucumber will do. If using a conventional cucumber with a waxy skin, you might prefer peeling and discarding the skin.*

....

....

Tip: *To slice herb leaves thinly quickly and without bruising them, stack the leaves in a neat pile, roll them up lengthwise, then slice them crosswise.*

....

For the pesto
   ¼ cup packed fresh basil leaves, thinly sliced
   ¼ cup packed fresh mint leaves, thinly sliced
   1 tablespoon roasted unsalted almonds, finely chopped
   ½ small garlic clove, finely chopped (¼ teaspoon)
   1½ tablespoons extra virgin olive oil
   ⅛ teaspoon kosher salt

For the skewers
   12 cherry tomatoes (4.25 ounces; scant 1 cup)
   12 bocconcini (mini mozzarella balls) (5.25 ounces; 1 cup)
   4 peach slices, cut into thirds (2⅛ ounces; scant ½ cup)
   1 ounce prosciutto, torn into 12 pieces (¼ cup packed)
   1 Persian cucumber (3 ounces), cut in half lengthwise, then cut
      crosswise into a total of 12 half-moon-shaped pieces
   12 fresh basil leaves (½ packed cup)

1. Prepare the pesto: In a blender, combine the basil, mint, almonds, garlic, oil, salt, and 2 tablespoons cold water and puree until smooth. Adjust the salt to taste.
2. Prepare the skewers: Thread 1 cherry tomato, 1 bocconcino, 1 peach piece, 1 prosciutto piece, 1 cucumber piece, and 1 basil leaf onto each of 12 skewers.
3. Drizzle with 2 tablespoons of pesto. Serve three skewers with a heaping teaspoon of pesto for dipping per person.

PER SERVING

ATKINS 100 • Net Carbs: 2 grams; Total Carbs: 4 grams; Fiber: 2 grams;
Protein: 10 grams; Fat: 17 grams; Calories: 200; FV: 1

RECIPES

ATKINS 20

ATKINS 40

ATKINS 100

CHAPTER 12

DESSERTS

Puddings and Pies, Plus Brownies and More

HOPEFULLY YOU'VE SAVED room for dessert! These sweet treats are the perfect ending to your low-carb meal. From cookies and cream to ice cream, these recipes are fruity, fresh, low carb, and guilt free!

The recipes in this chapter are categorized under Atkins 20, Atkins 40, and Atkins 100.

VANILLA BEAN EGG CUSTARD

SERVES 6 • TIME: *Active*—5 minutes *Total*—3 hours, including chilling

Here is a simple, classic egg custard, minus the sugar but just as good. You can easily vary it by adding citrus zest or swapping almond extract for the vanilla.

2 cups whole milk
2 large eggs
2 teaspoons vanilla extract
2 tablespoons stevia-erythritol blend
⅛ teaspoon kosher salt

1. Set an oven rack in the middle position. Preheat the oven to 350°F.
2. In a blender, blend all ingredients until smooth.
3. Divide the mixture among six 4-ounce ramekins or other heatproof cups. Place the ramekins in a baking dish and add hot tap water to come 1 inch up the sides of the cups.
4. Bake until the custards are just set, 35 to 45 minutes. Take the baking pan from the oven. Remove the ramekins from the water bath when cool enough to handle, then transfer to the refrigerator and chill until set, at least 2 hours or overnight.

PER SERVING

ATKINS 20 • Net Carbs: 4 grams; Total Carbs: 8 grams; Fiber: 0 grams;
Protein: 5 grams; Fat: 4 grams; Calories: 77; FV: 0

FLOURLESS DARK CHOCOLATE–CARDAMOM CAKE

SERVES 16 • TIME: *Active*—15 minutes *Total*—1 hour, 15 minutes,
including cooling • Makes one 8-inch cake

This rich, not-too-sweet cake more than satisfies a chocolate hankering. Made with antioxidant-rich unsweetened chocolate and cocoa powder, its fudgy center is part of the delight.

. . . .

Tip: A springform pan works best here, since you can easily release the sides once the cake is cooled. If you don't have one, a well-greased standard cake pan also works; just be gentle when turning the cake onto the plate.

. . . .

Olive oil spray
4 ounces unsweetened baking chocolate, chopped (scant 1 cup)
½ cup (1 stick) unsalted butter, cut into pieces

2 tablespoons stevia extract powder

¾ teaspoon ground cardamom

½ teaspoon ground cinnamon

¼ teaspoon kosher salt

4 large eggs

½ cup heavy cream

¼ cup unsweetened cocoa powder, plus more for dusting

1. Set an oven rack in the middle position. Preheat the oven to 350°F. Coat the bottom and sides of an 8-inch springform pan or standard cake pan with olive oil spray. Line the bottom with parchment paper and lightly coat the parchment paper with the spray.

2. In a large microwave safe bowl, combine the chocolate and butter and microwave on high in 20-second increments, stirring after each, until melted, about 1 minute 20 seconds total. (Alternatively, gently melt in a double boiler or in the top of two saucepans set up in a double-boiler style.)

3. Add the stevia, cardamom, cinnamon, and salt to the chocolate mixture and whisk to combine. Add the eggs and cream and whisk to combine, then whisk in the cocoa powder. Pour the batter into the prepared pan. Smooth with a rubber spatula. Bake until the cake has risen evenly, the edges are set, and a toothpick inserted into the center comes out mostly clean (the center will still be moist; do not overbake), 18 to 20 minutes.

4. Transfer the pan to a wire rack and let cool completely. Remove the sides of the pan (if using a springform pan) or carefully invert the cake onto a plate. Dust with cocoa powder and serve.

PER SERVING

ATKINS 20 • Net Carbs: 2 grams; Total Carbs: 4 grams; Fiber: 2 grams; Protein: 3 grams; Fat: 13 grams; Calories: 134; FV: 0

LOW-CARB DALGONA COFFEE

SERVES 8 • TIME: *Active*—15 minutes *Total*—15 minutes

This rich, creamy whipped coffee drink makes a delightful dessert. Regular or decaf instant coffee or espresso can be used.

. . . .

Tip: *The coffee foam can be beaten by hand with a whisk; it will take more time and a bit of arm muscle.*

. . . .

2 tablespoons instant coffee or espresso
2 tablespoons granulated erythritol
4 cups half-and-half

1. In a large bowl, beat the instant coffee powder, erythritol, and 2 tablespoons hot tap water with an electric mixer on medium-high speed until it is lightened in color and stiff peaks form, 4 to 7 minutes. You will have about 1½ cups of foam.
2. For each serving, fill an 8-ounce glass with ice and ½ cup half-and-half. Dollop 3 tablespoons of the coffee foam on top. Sip it as is, or stir to combine. The foam will keep, covered and refrigerated, for up to 2 days.

PER SERVING

ATKINS 20 • Net Carbs: 5 grams; Total Carbs: 8 grams; Protein: 3 grams; Fiber: 0 grams; Fat: 14 grams; Calories: 159; FV: 0

CREAMY COCONUT-COCOA ICE POPS

SERVES 4 • TIME: *Active*—10 minutes *Total*—6 hours, including freezing

This lightened-up version of the nostalgic ice cream truck Fudgsicle treat is delicious and fun to make. If you don't have ice pop molds, use small paper cups, such as Dixie cups. Divide the chocolate-coconut mixture among the cups, cover the tops with aluminum foil, then pierce a wooden pop stick through the foil (the foil keeps the sticks in place while the pops freeze). To eat, remove the foil and tear away the cup.

....

Tip: Coconut cream and coconut milk are often located next to each other at the grocery store, but they are not interchangeable; coconut cream is thicker and richer, and it's what gives these popsicles their creamy texture. Check the label to be sure you buy what you need.

....

1 (13-ounce) can unsweetened full-fat coconut cream
¼ cup unsweetened cocoa powder
2 tablespoons stevia-erythritol blend
1½ teaspoons vanilla extract
⅓ cup unsweetened shredded coconut

1. In a blender, combine the coconut cream, cocoa, stevia, and vanilla and puree until smooth, 20 to 30 seconds. Add the shredded coconut and pulse to combine, about 10 times. Divide the mixture among four ice pop molds and freeze for at least 6 hours.
2. To serve, run hot water over the mold, then slowly take out the ice pop. Let thaw 2 to 3 minutes before eating for the creamiest texture.

PER SERVING

ATKINS 20 • Net Carbs: 5 grams; Total Carbs: 13 grams; Fiber: 3 grams; Protein: 3 grams; Fat: 26 grams; Calories: 267; FV: 0

NO-CHURN MINT CHIP ICE CREAM

SERVES 8 • TIME: *Active*—15 minutes *Total*—6 hours, 15 minutes, including freezing

This creamy, mint-packed ice cream is made without the hassle of an ice cream maker. No-churn ice cream typically uses sweetened condensed milk, but we use evaporated milk and add a low-carb sweetener to keep this recipe sugar free. For the creamiest texture, let the ice cream thaw at room temperature for 5 to 10 minutes before scooping.

....
Tip: If you like a green mint chip ice cream, add a few drops of green food coloring to the cream before whipping.
....

1 (12-ounce) can evaporated milk
2 tablespoons stevia extract powder
2 teaspoons peppermint extract
½ teaspoon vanilla extract
2 cups heavy cream
3 ounces unsweetened chocolate, finely chopped (½ cup)

1. In a large bowl, stir together the evaporated milk, stevia, peppermint extract, and vanilla extract.
2. In a second large bowl, beat the cream with a hand or electric mixer on medium high until stiff peaks form, 3 to 4 minutes. Gently fold in the evaporated milk mixture and chocolate until well combined.
3. Transfer the ice cream base to a 6-cup freezer-safe pan or bowl and freeze until the ice cream is frozen solid, at least 6 hours.

PER SERVING
ATKINS 40 • Net Carbs: 8 grams; Total Carbs: 10 grams; Fiber: 2 grams; Protein: 6 grams; Fat: 30 grams; Calories: 322; FV: 0

BERRIES WITH LEMON CASHEW CREAM

SERVES 4 • TIME: *Active*—20 minutes *Total*—12 hours

Protein-packed cashew cream is a great vegan replacement for conventional whipped cream and delightful atop juicy, antioxidant-rich berries. Soaking the cashews overnight allows them to blend to a silky-smooth consistency, so be sure to start this recipe one day ahead. Tossing the berries in lemon juice and a pinch of stevia draws out their juices to create a sweet, fruity syrup. It's extra-delicious when berries are at their peak.

....

Tip: Any combination of blueberries, raspberries, and blackberries can be used. Just be sure to adjust the carb count accordingly.

....

For the cashew cream
   ¾ cup raw, unsalted cashews (3¼ ounces)
   1 teaspoon lemon zest
   1 tablespoon fresh lemon juice
   ½ teaspoon vanilla extract
   ⅛ teaspoon stevia powder

For the berries
   1 cup raspberries, washed and patted dry
   ½ cup blueberries, washed and patted dry
   ½ cup blackberries, washed and patted dry
   1 tablespoon fresh lemon juice
   ½ teaspoon stevia extract powder
   Lemon zest, for garnish

1. Prepare the cashew cream: In a medium bowl, combine the cashews and 2 cups of tepid water. Let stand uncovered at room temperature until the cashews break apart easily when pressed between two fingers, 10 to 12 hours.

2. Drain the cashews and discard the soaking water. In a blender, combine the drained cashews, lemon zest, lemon juice, vanilla extract, stevia, and ¼ cup tepid water. Blend on high speed, stopping after every minute to scrape down the sides, until smooth, about 3 minutes. The cashew cream can be made up to 1 week ahead. Store, covered, in the refrigerator until ready to serve.

3. Macerate the berries: In a medium bowl, gently stir together the raspberries, blueberries, blackberries, lemon juice, and stevia. Set aside until the berries begin to release some of their juices, at least 1 hour at room temperature or in the refrigerator for up to 1 day.

4. Divide the berries among four serving bowls, a scant ½ cup per bowl. Top each with about 3 tablespoons of the cashew cream and the lemon zest and serve.

PER SERVING

ATKINS 40 • Net Carbs: 9 grams; Total Carbs: 15 grams; Fiber: 6 grams;
   Protein: 5 grams; Fat: 11 grams; Calories: 175; FV: 0

CHERRIES AND CREAM

SERVES 6 • TIME: *Active*—25 minutes *Total*—25 minutes

Low-carb cherries combine with orange peel and fresh orange juice to create a naturally sweet and super-simple compote to spoon over the rich and creamy yogurt. Finish each serving with chopped pistachios for color and crunch.

> ....
> **Tip:** *To create strips of orange peel, use a sharp Y-shaped or*
> *regular vegetable peeler to create four 1- to 2-inch-wide strips of*
> *peel, removing as little of the white pith as possible as you go.*
> ....

¼ cup salted, shelled pistachios (1 ounce)
2 cups plain full-fat Greek yogurt
1 teaspoon vanilla extract
1½ cups frozen dark sweet cherries (7.5 ounces)
4 strips orange peel
1 tablespoon fresh orange juice
4 whole star anise

1. Preheat the oven to 350°F. Place the pistachios on a baking sheet. Bake until fragrant and lightly golden, about 5 minutes. Transfer to a plate and let cool completely, then finely chop.
2. In a medium bowl, stir together the yogurt and vanilla extract and set aside.
3. In a medium saucepan, add the cherries, orange peel, orange juice, and star anise and cook over medium heat, stirring occasionally, until the mixture begins to simmer, then reduce to medium low. Continue cooking until the cherries are softened and the juices thicken to a pourable glaze, 8 to 10 minutes. Remove and discard the orange peel and star anise.
4. Arrange ½ cup yogurt and ¼ cup cherry mixture in each of four serving bowls. Drizzle any remaining juices over the top. Top each serving with 1 heaping tablespoon of pistachios.

PER SERVING

ATKINS 40 • Net Carbs: 9 grams; Total Carbs: 10 grams; Fiber: 1 gram; Protein: 9 grams; Fat: 7 grams; Calories: 401; FV: 0

FLOURLESS SALTED PEANUT BUTTER CHOCOLATE CHIP COOKIES

MAKES 24 COOKIES • TIME: *Active*—40 minutes *Total*—50 minutes, plus cooling

These gluten-free cookies unite the beloved classic combo: chocolate and protein-packed peanut butter. No fancy equipment is needed: the criss-cross chocolate drizzle is easy to do with a fork. A sprinkling of flaky sea salt takes these tasty treats over the top.

. . . .

Tip: *If you're using a brand of peanut butter that separates, stir it thoroughly until smooth before making the cookies.*

. . . .

1 cup sugar-free smooth or creamy peanut butter
2 teaspoons stevia extract powder
½ teaspoon baking soda
¼ teaspoon kosher salt
1 large egg
1 teaspoon vanilla extract
½ cup sugar-free semisweet chocolate chips
1 teaspoon flaky sea salt, such as Maldon

1. Set oven racks in the upper and lower third positions. Preheat the oven to 350°F. Line two cookie sheets with parchment paper.
2. In a medium bowl, beat the peanut butter, stevia, baking soda, and salt with a handheld electric mixer on medium speed, scraping down the sides if needed, until well combined, about 1 minute. Reduce the speed to low, add the egg and vanilla extract, and beat until combined.
3. Shape the dough into 24 balls (scant 1 tablespoon each) and place 2 inches apart on the prepared cookie sheets. Using the tines of a fork,

carefully flatten each ball, creating a crisscross pattern. (Dampen the fork with water if it sticks.)

4. Bake, rotating the cookie sheets from top to bottom and from back to front halfway through, until the edges are just beginning to brown and the cookies are just set, 7 to 9 minutes. (Do not overbake; the cookies should not be browned.) Let cool for 10 minutes on the cookie sheet, then carefully transfer to a cooling rack to cool completely.

5. In a small microwave-safe bowl, add the chocolate chips and microwave on high in 20-second increments, stirring after each, until melted, about 1 minute total. (Alternatively, gently melt in a double boiler or in the top of two saucepans set up in a double-boiler style.)

6. Dip a dry fork into the chocolate, then drizzle the chocolate over the cookies. Sprinkle with sea salt. Serve 1 cookie per person.

PER SERVING

ATKINS 40 • Net Carbs: 1.5 grams; Total Carbs: 3 grams; Fiber: 1.5 grams; Protein: 3 grams; Fat: 6.5 grams; Calories: 79; FV: 0

CHOCOLATE-HAZELNUT BROWNIE BITES

MAKES 18 BITES • TIME: *Active*—10 minutes *Total*—35 minutes, plus cooling time

Nutella fans, rejoice! These gluten-free bites are packed with chocolate-hazelnut flavor, thanks to vitamin-rich hazelnut meal and 100 percent chocolate, which is low in carbs and rich in heart-healthy flavonoids. A sprinkling of flaky sea salt brings out the intense chocolatey flavor. Easy to transport, these treats are great for bake sales, potlucks, and lunch box snacks. Unused portions freeze beautifully and warm easily; they're great to have on hand when you want a sweet treat.

··································

Tip: *Hazelnut meal and hazelnut flour are the same product and can be used interchangeably.*

··································

Tip: *Due to their high oil content, nut and other alternative flours tend to go rancid faster than their wheat counterparts. To extend their shelf life, store them in the refrigerator or freezer.*

··································

Olive oil spray

4 ounces unsweetened chocolate, chopped (¾ cup)

½ cup (1 stick) unsalted butter

¼ cup plain unsweetened almond milk

4 large eggs

2 teaspoons vanilla extract

½ cup granulated erythritol

1 teaspoon stevia extract powder

¼ cup hazelnut meal or flour (1 ounce)

2 tablespoons unsweetened cocoa powder

1 teaspoon baking powder

¼ teaspoon flaky sea salt, such as Maldon

1. Set an oven rack in the middle position. Preheat the oven to 350°F. Coat a 9-by-13-inch cake pan with olive oil spray.

2. In a microwave-safe bowl, combine the chocolate, butter, and almond milk and microwave on high in 30-second increments, stirring after each, until the chocolate is melted, about 2 minutes total. (Alternatively, gently melt in a double boiler or in the top of two saucepans set up double-boiler style.) Set aside to cool completely, 10 to 12 minutes.

3. Add the eggs and vanilla extract to the cooled chocolate mixture and beat to combine.

4. In a large bowl, whisk together the erythritol, stevia, hazelnut meal, cocoa powder, and baking powder to combine. Stir in the chocolate mixture just to combine.

5. Transfer the batter to the prepared pan. Smooth the top with a rubber spatula. Sprinkle with sea salt. Bake until the edges are firm but the center is still soft, 18 to 22 minutes. Cool a bit in the pan, then cut into 18 pieces. For the best flavor, serve warm.

6. The bites will keep, covered and at cool room temperature, for up to 5 days or frozen for up to 2 months. Warm in a 200°F oven for 5 to 10 minutes before serving. If frozen, thaw at room temperature before warming.

PER SERVING

ATKINS 100 • Net Carbs: 7 grams; Total Carbs: 8 grams; Fiber: 1 gram; Protein: 3 grams; Fat: 10 grams; Calories: 106; FV: 0

CHOCOLATE-RASPBERRY BREAD PUDDING

SERVES 10 • TIME: *Active*—20 minutes *Total*—2 hours, 30 minutes

Can bread pudding go hand in hand with a low-carb lifestyle? Yes, it can! After soaking in a vanilla-flavored egg custard, low-carb bread bakes into a decadent dessert with the tender, fluffy texture we all know and love. Antioxidant-packed chocolate and raspberries make it that much better.

> **Tip:** *Look for low-carb bread, such as Base Culture Original Keto Bread, in the freezer aisle of your grocery store. Low-carb bread is denser than standard bread. The longer it sits in the custard, the more tender your pudding will be. Let it soak as long as one day, if you have time to prepare the pudding ahead.*

Olive oil spray

1½ cups heavy cream

6 large eggs

¼ cup granulated sucralose-based sweetener

2 teaspoons stevia extract powder

2 teaspoons vanilla extract

¼ teaspoon kosher salt

8 slices low-carb bread, such as Base Culture Original Keto Bread,
*   thawed and cut into 1-inch cubes (about 8 cups)*

½ cup (3 ounces) sugar-free semisweet dark chocolate chips

½ cup fresh raspberries

1. Lightly coat an 8½-by-4½-inch loaf pan with olive oil spray. In a large bowl, whisk together the cream, eggs, sucralose-based sweetener, stevia, vanilla extract, salt, and 2 tablespoons tepid water to combine.

2. Arrange half each of the bread cubes, chocolate chips, and raspberries in the prepared pan. Top with the remaining bread, then pour the cream mixture over the top. Press the bread with the back of a large spoon to fully submerge it in the liquid. Sprinkle with the remaining chocolate chips and raspberries.

3. Let the mixture stand until the cream mixture fully soaks into the bread, at least 1 hour at room temperature or up to 24 hours in the refrigerator.

4. Set an oven rack in the middle position. Preheat the oven to 300°F.

5. Place the loaf pan into a larger baking pan and fill the baking pan with boiling water to come halfway up the sides.

6. Bake until the bread pudding is puffed up, golden on top, and springy but firm when pressed and an instant-read thermometer inserted in the center reads 160°F, 65 to 75 minutes.

7. Serve a heaping ½ cupful of bread pudding per person, warm or at room temperature.

PER SERVING

Atkins 100 • Net Carbs: 8 grams; Total Carbs: 15 grams; Fiber: 7 grams;
Protein: 8 grams; Fat: 24 grams; Calories: 292; FV: 0

FRESH PEACH AND CINNAMON NO-CHURN ICE CREAM

SERVES 8 • TIME: *Active*—15 minutes *Total*—6 hours, 25 minutes,
including freezing

Sweet chunks of high-fiber peaches add a pop of juicy fruit to every bite of this creamy ice cream. A touch of cinnamon makes for a surprisingly delicious combo.

....

Tip: When peaches are in season, look for ones that are free of blemishes and give slightly when gently pressed. During winter months, substitute thawed frozen peaches.

....

1 (12-ounce) can evaporated milk
1½ tablespoons stevia extract powder
1 teaspoon ground cinnamon
1 teaspoon vanilla extract
2 cups coarsely chopped fresh or thawed frozen peaches
2 cups heavy cream

1. In a blender, blend the evaporated milk, stevia, cinnamon, and vanilla extract until smooth. Add the peaches and pulse a few times to further chop and incorporate the fruit.
2. In a large bowl, whisk the cream with a hand whisk or an electric hand mixer on medium high until stiff peaks form, 3 to 4 minutes. Gently fold in the peach mixture until completely combined.

3. Transfer the ice cream base to an 8-cup freezer-safe pan or bowl and freeze until the ice cream is frozen solid, at least 6 hours.

4. Let the ice cream thaw at room temperature for 5 to 10 minutes before scooping for the creamiest texture. Serve ¾ cup per person.

PER SERVING

ATKINS 100 • Net Carbs: 10 grams; Total Carbs: 11 grams; Fiber: 1 gram; Protein: 5 grams; Fat: 25 grams; Calories: 282; FV: 0

PUMPKIN PIE AND TOASTED WALNUT "NICE CREAM"

SERVES 4 • TIME: *Active*—15 minutes *Total*—2 hours. 20 minutes

Making "ice cream" with frozen bananas is magic: in mere minutes they transform in the food processor from frozen to crumbly to impossibly smooth. Adding pumpkin puree and pumpkin pie spice gives this treat the flavor of a slice of rich pumpkin pie. Walnuts, which are packed with antioxidants and omega-3 fats, add a wonderful crunch.

....

Tip: *A blend of cinnamon and nutmeg can be used in place of pumpkin pie spice.*

....

Tip: *Pumpkin puree (which is unsweetened) and pumpkin pie filling (which contains sugar and other added ingredients) can be easily confused at the market. Be sure to use the former. Leftover puree can be frozen for up to three months.*

....

2 small bananas, sliced (6.5 ounces peeled, 1½ cups sliced)
3 tablespoons unsweetened pumpkin puree
3 tablespoons walnut halves and pieces

½ teaspoon pumpkin pie spice

¼ teaspoon almond extract

⅛ teaspoon stevia extract powder

1. Place the bananas and pumpkin puree in a resealable freezer bag with the air pressed out, then seal and freeze until frozen solid, at least 2 hours or (ideally) overnight.
2. Preheat the oven to 350°F.
3. Spread the walnuts on a baking sheet and bake until fragrant and lightly toasted, 5 to 7 minutes. Let cool completely, then chop coarsely.
4. Just before you're ready to serve, in a food processor fitted with the blade attachment, process the frozen banana mixture until crumbled, about 1 minute. Add the pumpkin pie spice, almond extract, and stevia. Continue processing until completely smooth, 1 to 2 minutes more.
5. Transfer the "nice cream" to a medium bowl. Working quickly, fold in the chopped walnuts, then scoop ¼ cup plus 2 tablespoons into each of four serving bowls and serve immediately.

PER SERVING

ATKINS 100 • Net Carbs: 10 grams; Total Carbs: 12 grams; Fiber: 2 grams; Protein: 2 grams; Fat: 4 grams; Calories: 85; FV: 0

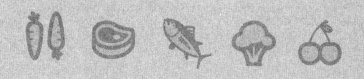

ATKINS 20, LEVEL 1, ACCEPTABLE FOODS

This is an extensive list, but it may not include all possible acceptable foods.

FISH AND SHELLFISH

Most fish and shellfish contain no carbs. All are acceptable with the following exceptions:

- Pickled herring prepared with sugar, artificial crab (surimi), sold as "sea legs," and other processed shellfish products
- Oysters and mussels; these contain carbs, so limit your consumption of them to about 4 ounces per day
- Breaded seafood

POULTRY

All pure poultry products are acceptable. Do not use any products with breading or fillers.

MEAT

All pure meat products are acceptable. Avoid processed meats with fillers (some salami, pepperoni, hog dogs, meatballs), breaded, or cured with sugar (bacon, ham).

EGGS

Eggs prepared in any style are acceptable.

SOY AND VEGETARIAN PRODUCTS

- Quorn products contain milk and eggs, making them unsuitable for vegans.
- Soy cheeses that contain casein, a milk product, are also unsuitable for vegans.
- Many veggie burgers have carb counts higher than 2 grams of Net Carbs and ingredients that may not be acceptable in Level 1.

	Serving Size	Grams of Net Carbs
Almond milk, unsweetened	1 cup	1.0
Quorn burger	1 burger	4.0
Quorn cutlet, unbreaded	1 cutlet	3.0
Quorn roast	4 ounces	4.0
Seitan	1 piece	2.0
Shirataki soy noodles	½ cup cooked	1.0
Soy "cheese"	1 slice	1.0
Soy "cheese"	1 ounce	2.0
Soy milk, plain, unsweetened	8 ounces	1.2
Tempeh	½ cup	3.3
Tofu, firm	4 ounces	2.5
Tofu, silken, soft	4 ounces	3.1
Tofu "bacon"	2 strips	2.0
Tofu "Canadian bacon"	3 slices	1.5
Tofu "hot dogs"	1 "hot dog"	2.0–5.0, depending on brand
Tofu "sausage," bulk	2 ounces	2.0

Tofu "sausage," links	2 links	4.0
Vegan "cheese," no casein	1 slice	5.0
Vegan "cheese," no casein	1 ounce	6.0
Veggie burger	1 burger	2.0
Veggie crumbles	⅓ cup	2.0
Veggie "meatballs"	4–5 balls	4.0

Note: Check individual products for exact carb counts.

CHEESE

All cheese except ricotta and cottage cheese (they can be added in Level 2) is acceptable. Note the following:

- You may eat up to 4 ounces a day. A tablespoon or two of any grated cheese contains a negligible number of carbs.
- Avoid cheese spreads that contain other ingredients (strawberry-flavored cream cheese, for example), "diet" cheese, "cheese products," and whey cheeses, none of which is 100 percent cheese.
- Soy or rice "cheese" is acceptable, but check the carb count.

FOUNDATION VEGETABLES

These include both salad vegetables and others that are usually cooked.

Salad Vegetables

- Measure the following salad vegetables raw (except for artichoke hearts).
- Tomatoes, onions, and bell peppers are higher in carbs than other salad vegetables, so use them in smaller portions.
- Included in this list are fruits generally thought of as vegetables, such as avocados and olives.

	Serving Size	Grams of Net Carbs
Alfalfa sprouts	½ cup	0.2
Artichoke hearts, canned	1 heart	1.0
Artichoke hearts, marinated	4 pieces	2.0
Arugula	1 cup	0.4
Avocado, Haas	½ avocado	1.8
Beans, green, snap, string, or wax	½ cup	2.1
Bok choy (pak choi), shredded	1 cup	0.4
Boston/Bibb lettuce, shredded	1 cup	0.8
Broccoli florets	½ cup	0.8
Cabbage, green, red, Savoy, shredded	½ cup	1.1
Cauliflower florets	½ cup	1.4
Celery	1 stalk	0.8
Celery root (celeriac), grated	½ cup	3.5
Chicory greens	½ cup	0.1
Chinese cabbage, shredded	½ cup	0.0
Chives	1 tablespoon	0.1
Cucumber	½ cup	1.0
Daikon radish, chopped	½ cup	1.0
Endive, chopped	½ cup	0.4
Escarole, shredded	½ cup	0.1
Fennel	½ cup	1.8
Greens, mixed	1 cup	0.4
Iceberg lettuce, shredded	1 cup	0.2
Jicama, chopped	½ cup	2.5
Loose-leaf lettuce	1 cup	1.0
Mesclun	1 cup	0.5

Mung bean sprouts	½ cup	2.1
Mushrooms, button, fresh	½ cup	1.2
Olives, black	5 olives	0.7
Olives, green	5 olives	0.0
Onion, chopped	2 tablespoons	0.5
Parsley (and all other fresh herbs), chopped	1 tablespoon	0.1
Pepper, green bell, chopped	½ cup	2.1
Pepper, red bell, chopped	½ cup	2.9
Radicchio	½ cup	0.7
Radishes	6 radishes	0.5
Rhubarb, unsweetened, chopped	½ cup	1.7
Romaine lettuce	1 cup	0.4
Scallions, chopped	¼ cup	1.2
Spinach	1 cup	0.2
Tomato	1 small tomato (3–4 ounces)	2.5
Tomato	1 medium tomato	3.3
Tomato, cherry	5 tomatoes	2.2
Watercress	½ cup	0.0

Cooked Vegetables

- Some of these also appear on the salad vegetables list, but cooking compacts them, which explains the differences in carb counts.
- Some vegetables, such as celery root, kohlrabi, leeks, mushrooms, onions, and pumpkin, are higher in carbs than most, which accounts for the smaller portions.
- Vegetables *not* on this list should not be consumed in Level 1.

	Serving Size	Grams of Net Carbs
Artichoke	½ medium	3.5
Asparagus	6 spears	2.4
Bamboo shoots, canned, sliced	½ cup	1.2
Beans, green, wax, string, or snap	½ cup	2.9
Beet greens	½ cup	3.7
Bok choy (pak choi)	½ cup	0.2
Broccoflower	½ cup	2.3
Broccoli	½ cup	1.7
Broccoli rabe	½ cup	2.0
Brussels sprouts	¼ cup	1.8
Cabbage, green	½ cup	1.6
Cabbage, red	½ cup	2.0
Cabbage, Savoy	½ cup	1.9
Cardoon	½ cup	2.7
Cauliflower	½ cup	0.9
Celery	½ cup	1.2
Chard, Swiss	½ cup	1.8
Chayote	½ cup	1.8
Collard greens	½ cup	2.0
Dandelion greens	½ cup	1.8
Eggplant	½ cup	2.0
Escarole	½ cup	0.1
Fennel	½ cup	1.5
Hearts of palm	1 heart	0.7
Kale	½ cup	2.4
Kohlrabi	¼ cup	2.3
Leeks	½ cup	3.4
Mushrooms, button	¼ cup	2.3

Mushrooms, shiitake	¼ cup	4.4
Mustard greens	½ cup	0.1
Nopales (cactus pads)	½ cup	1.0
Okra	½ cup	2.4
Onion	¼ cup	4.3
Pepper, green bell, chopped	¼ cup	1.9
Pepper, red bell, chopped	¼ cup	1.9
Pumpkin	¼ cup	2.4
Rhubarb, unsweetened	½ cup	1.7
Sauerkraut, drained	½ cup	1.2
Scallions	½ cup	2.4
Shallots	2 tablespoons	3.1
Snow peas/snap peas in the pod	½ cup	3.4
Sorrel	½ cup	0.2
Spaghetti squash	¼ cup	2.0
Spinach	½ cup	2.2
Summer squash	½ cup	2.6
Tomatillo	½ cup	2.6
Tomato	¼ cup	4.3
Turnips (white), mashed	½ cup	3.3
Water chestnuts, canned	¼ cup	3.5
Zucchini	½ cup	1.5

SALAD DRESSINGS

Any salad dressing with no more than 2 grams of Net Carbs per 2-tablespoon serving is acceptable. Note the following:

- Do *not* use sugar, honey, maple syrup, or other caloric sweeteners in salad dressings.

FATS AND OILS

Butter, canola oil, coconut oil, flaxseed oil, grape seed oil, olive oil, high-oleic safflower oil, sesame oil, and walnut oil are acceptable. Note the following:

- Oils labeled "cold pressed" or "expeller pressed" are preferable.
- Mayonnaise should be made with olive, canola, or high-oleic safflower oil.
- Use extra-virgin olive oil for dressing salad and vegetables and sautéing.
- Use olive, canola, or high-oleic safflower oil for other cooking.
- Use walnut, sesame, or other specialty oil to season a dish after removing it from the heat.
- Avoid products labeled "lite" or "low fat" and all margarines and shortening products, which still contain small amounts of trans fats.
- Avoid corn, soy, sunflower seed, and other vegetable oils.

NONCALORIC SWEETENERS

The following are acceptable in moderation: Splenda (sucralose), Swerve (erythritol), Truvia (erythritol-stevia blend), SweetLeaf (stevia), Sweet'N Low (saccharin), xylitol.

CONDIMENTS, HERBS, AND SPICES

All herbs, spices, and seasonings are acceptable. Note the following:

- Avoid any herb or spice mixture that contains added sugar.
- Avoid condiments made with sugar, flour, cornstarch, and other carb-filled thickeners.

The following products are acceptable:

	Serving Size	Grams of Net Carbs
Ancho chile pepper	1 pepper	5.1
Anchovy paste	1 tablespoon	0.0

Black bean sauce	1 teaspoon	3.0
Capers	1 tablespoon	0.1
Chipotle in adobe	2 peppers	2.0
Clam juice	1 cup	0.0
Enchilada sauce	¼ cup	2.0
Fish sauce	1 teaspoon	0.2
Garlic	1 large clove	0.9
Ginger root, grated	1 tablespoon	0.8
Horseradish sauce	1 teaspoon	0.4
Jalapeño pepper	½ cup sliced	1.4
Miso paste	1 tablespoon	2.6
Mustard, Dijon	1 teaspoon	0.5
Mustard, yellow	1 teaspoon	0.0
Olives, black	5 olives	0.7
Olives, green	5 olives	2.5
Pasilla chile pepper	1 pepper	1.7
Pesto sauce	1 tablespoon	0.6
Pickapeppa sauce	1 teaspoon	1.0
Pickle, dill or kosher	½ pickle	1.0
Pimento/roasted red pepper	1 ounce	2.0
Salsa, green, no added sugar	1 tablespoon	0.6
Salsa, red, no added sugar	1 tablespoon	1.0
Serrano chile pepper	½ cup	1.6
Soy sauce	1 tablespoon	0.9
Tabasco or other hot sauce	1 teaspoon	0.0
Taco sauce	1 tablespoon	1.0
Tahini (sesame paste)	2 tablespoons	1.0
Vinegar, balsamic	1 tablespoon	2.3
Vinegar, cider	1 tablespoon	0.9

Vinegar, red wine	1 tablespoon	1.5
Vinegar, rice, unsweetened	1 tablespoon	0.0
Vinegar, sherry	1 tablespoon	0.9
Vinegar, white wine	1 tablespoon	1.5
Wasabi paste	1 teaspoon	0.0

BEVERAGES

The following beverages are acceptable:
- Broth/bouillon
- Club soda
- Coffee or tea, caffeinated or decaffeinated
- Cream, heavy or light, or half-and-half, 1 to 1.5 ounces a day
- Diet soda sweetened with noncaloric sweeteners
- Herb tea without added barley or fruit sugar
- Lemon juice or lime juice; limit to 2 to 3 tablespoons a day
- Seltzer, plain or essence-flavored (must say "no calories")
- Soy or almond milk, unsweetened and unflavored

ATKINS 20, LEVEL 2, ACCEPTABLE FOODS

In addition to the acceptable foods for Level 1, the following are acceptable in Level 2.

NUTS AND SEEDS AND THEIR BUTTERS

Most nuts and seeds and butters made from them are acceptable. Note the following:

- Consume no more than 2 ounces (about ¼ cup) a day.
- Nut meals and flours broaden your cooking options.
- Avoid honey-roasted and smoked products.
- Chestnuts are very starchy and high in carbs, making them unsuitable for this level.
- Avoid products such as Nutella that include sugar or other sweeteners.

The following list provides portion sizes equivalent to 1 ounce:

	Serving Size	Grams of Net Carbs
Almond butter	1 tablespoon	2.5
Almond meal/flour	¼ cup	3.0
Almonds	24 nuts	2.3
Brazil nuts	5 nuts	2.0
Cashew butter	1 tablespoon	4.1
Cashews	9 nuts	4.4
Coconut, shredded, unsweetened	¼ cup	1.3
Hazelnuts	12 nuts	0.5
Macadamia butter	1 tablespoon	2.5
Macadamia nuts	6 nuts	2.0
Peanut butter, natural	1 tablespoon	2.4
Peanut butter, smooth	1 tablespoon	2.2
Peanuts	22 nuts	1.5
Pecans	10 halves	1.5
Pine nuts (piñons)	2 tablespoons	1.7
Pistachios	25 nuts	2.5
Pumpkin seeds, hulled	2 tablespoons	2.0
Sesame seeds	2 tablespoons	1.6
Soy "nut" butter	1 tablespoon	3.0
Soy "nuts"	2 tablespoons	2.7
Sunflower seed butter	1 tablespoon	0.5
Sunflower seeds, hulled	2 tablespoons	1.1
Tahini (sesame paste)	1 tablespoon	0.8
Walnuts	7 halves	1.5

BERRIES AND OTHER FRUITS

All berries are acceptable, as are melon (except watermelon) and cherries. Note the following:

- All fruits should be regarded as garnishes, not major components of a dish.
- Also acceptable are small (1-tablespoon) portions of preserves made without added sugar. Each tablespoon should provide no more than 2 grams of Net Carbs.

	Serving Size	Grams of Net Carbs
Blackberries, fresh	¼ cup	2.7
Blackberries, frozen	¼ cup	4.1
Blueberries, fresh	¼ cup	4.1
Blueberries, frozen	¼ cup	3.7
Boysenberries, fresh	¼ cup	2.7
Boysenberries, frozen	¼ cup	2.8
Cherries, sour, fresh	¼ cup	2.8
Cherries, sweet, fresh	¼ cup	4.2
Cranberries, raw	¼ cup	2.0
Currants, fresh	¼ cup	2.5
Gooseberries, fresh	½ cup	4.4
Loganberries, fresh	¼ cup	2.7
Melon, cantaloupe, balls	¼ cup	3.7
Melon, Crenshaw, balls	¼ cup	2.3
Melon, honeydew, balls	¼ cup	3.6
Raspberries, fresh	¼ cup	1.5
Raspberries, frozen	¼ cup	1.8
Strawberries, fresh	1 large	1.0
Strawberries, fresh, sliced	¼ cup	1.8
Strawberries, frozen	¼ cup	2.6

FRESH CHEESE AND OTHER DAIRY PRODUCTS

You may now reintroduce the remaining fresh cheeses. Note the following:

- Use only plain, unsweetened, whole-milk yogurt or Greek yogurt.
- Avoid processed yogurt made with fruit or other flavorings or added sugar.
- Avoid low-fat and no-fat cottage cheese and yogurt products.

	Serving Size	Grams of Net Carbs
Cheese, cottage, full fat	½ cup	2.8
Cheese, cottage, 2% fat	½ cup	4.1
Milk, whole, evaporated	2 tablespoons	3.0
Ricotta, whole milk	½ cup	3.8
Yogurt, Greek, whole milk, plain, unsweetened	4 ounces	3.5
Yogurt, plain, low carb	4 ounces	3.0
Yogurt, whole milk, plain, unsweetened	4 ounces	5.5

LEGUMES

- Use small portions, and regard legumes as a garnish.
- Avoid baked beans, which are full of sugar, and other products such as beans in tomato sauce with sugar or starches and bean dips.
- Black soybeans are far lower in carbs than black (or turtle) beans with no trade-off in taste.

The serving sizes for dried and fresh legumes are the same, but the serving size for dried legumes are for after they are cooked, and the serving size for fresh legumes are for shelled beans.

	Serving Size	Grams of Net Carbs
Beans, black or turtle	¼ cup	6.5
Beans, cannellini	¼ cup	8.5
Beans, cranberry/Roman	¼ cup	6.3
Beans, fava	¼ cup	6.0
Beans, Great Northern	¼ cup	6.3
Beans, kidney	¼ cup	5.8
Beans, Lima, baby	¼ cup	7.1
Beans, Lima, large	¼ cup	6.5
Beans, navy	¼ cup	9.1
Beans, pink	¼ cup	9.6
Beans, pinto	¼ cup	7.3
Beans, refried, canned	¼ cup	6.5
Chickpeas/garbanzo beans	¼ cup	6.5
Hummus, plain	2 tablespoons	4.6
Lentils	¼ cup	6.0
Peas, black-eyed	¼ cup	6.2
Peas, pigeon	¼ cup	7.0
Peas, split	¼ cup	6.3
Soybeans, black	½ cup	1.0
Soybeans, green edamame	¼ cup	3.1

VEGETABLE AND FRUIT JUICES

- Most fruit juices are completely off limits.
- In Level 2, you can double the amount of lemon and lime juice.
- You can now also introduce small portions of tomato juice or tomato juice cocktail.

	Serving Size	Grams of Net Carbs
Lemon juice	¼ cup	5.2
Lime juice	¼ cup	5.6
Tomato juice	4 ounces	4.2
Tomato juice cocktail	4 ounces	4.5

LOW-CARB PRODUCTS

In each case, we've provided the *maximum* acceptable carb count for a single serving. If the carb count of a specific product exceeds the amount listed below, pass it up.

	Serving Size	Maximum Grams of Net Carbs
Atkins Flour Mix (page 197)	¾ cup	5.0
Bagels, low carb	1 bagel	5.0
Bread, low carb	1 slice	6.0
Chocolate/candy, low carb	1.2 ounces	3.0
Dairy drink, low carb	8 ounces	4.0
Ice cream, no added sugar	½ cup	4.0
Pancakes, low carb	2 pancakes	6.0
Pita, low carb, 6 inch	1 pita	4.0
Rolls, low carb	1 roll	4.0
Soy chips, low carb	1 ounce	5.0
Tortillas, low carb, 7 inch	1 tortilla	4.0

ATKINS 20, LEVELS 3 AND 4, ACCEPTABLE FOODS

In addition to all the foods you can eat in Levels 1 and 2, the following foods are acceptable in Levels 3 and 4.

FRUITS OTHER THAN BERRIES

- All fruit is high in sugar and should be treated as a garnish.
- Avoid canned fruit, even packed in juice concentrate or "lite" syrup.
- Continue to avoid fruit juice, other than lemon and lime juice.
- Avoid dried fruit.

The following carb counts are for fresh fruit:

	Serving Size	Grams of Net Carbs
Apple	½ medium	8.7
Apricot	3 medium	9.2
Banana	1 small	21.2
Carambola (star fruit), sliced	½ cup	2.8
Cherimoya, sliced	½ cup	24.3

Fig	1 small	6.4
Grapefruit, red	½ medium	7.9
Grapefruit, white	½ medium	8.6
Grapes, Concord	½ cup	7.4
Grapes, green	½ cup	13.7
Grapes, red	½ cup	13.4
Guava, sliced	½ cup	5.3
Kiwi	1 medium	8.7
Kumquat	4 medium	7.5
Loquat	10 medium	14.2
Lychees	½ cup	14.5
Mango, sliced	½ cup	12.5
Nectarine	1 medium	13.8
Orange	1 medium	12.9
Orange, sections	½ cup	8.4
Papaya	½ small	6.1
Passion fruit	¼ cup	7.7
Peach	1 small	7.2
Pear, Bartlett	1 medium	21.1
Pear, Bosc	1 small	17.7
Persimmon	½ medium	12.6
Pineapple, chunks	½ cup	8.7
Plantain	½ cup	21.0
Plum	½ small	3.3
Pomegranate	¼ medium	6.4
Quince	1 medium	12.3
Tangerine	1 medium	6.2
Watermelon, balls	½ cup	5.1

STARCHY VEGETABLES

All vegetables are measured after cooking except for Jerusalem artichoke.

	Serving Size	Grams of Net Carbs
Artichoke, Jerusalem	½ cup	11.9
Beets	½ cup	6.8
Burdock	½ cup	12.1
Calabaza (Spanish pumpkin), mashed	½ cup	5.9
Carrot	1 medium	5.6
Cassava (yuca), mashed	½ cup	25.1
Corn	½ cup	12.6
Corn on the cob	1 ear	17.2
Parsnips	½ cup	10.5
Potato, small, baked	½ potato	10.5
Rutabaga	½ cup	5.9
Squash, acorn, baked	½ cup	7.8
Squash, acorn, steamed	½ cup	7.6
Squash, butternut, baked	½ cup	7.9
Sweet potato, baked	½ potato	12.1
Taro	½ cup	19.5
Yam, sliced	½ cup	16.1
Yautia (arracacha), sliced	½ cup	29.9

WHOLE GRAINS

- Avoid refined grains, such as white flour, "enriched flour," and white rice.
- Baked goods should be made with 100 percent whole grains.

	Serving Size	Grams of Net Carbs
Barley, hulled, cooked	½ cup	13.0
Barley, pearled, cooked	½ cup	19.0
Bulgur wheat, cooked	½ cup	12.8
Cornmeal	2 tablespoons	10.6
Couscous, cooked	½ cup	17.1
Cracked wheat, cooked	½ cup	15.0
Hominy, cooked	½ cup	9.7
Kasha (buckwheat groats), cooked	½ cup	14.0
Millet, cooked	½ cup	19.5
Oat bran	2 tablespoons	6.0
Oatmeal, rolled	⅓ cup	19.0
Oatmeal, steel cut, cooked	¼ cup	19.0
Quinoa, cooked	¼ cup	27.0
Rice, brown, cooked	½ cup	20.5
Rice, wild, cooked	½ cup	16.0
Wheat berries, cooked	½ cup	14.0

DAIRY PRODUCTS

- You can also add small portions of whole milk (4 ounces contain almost 6 grams of Net Carbs) or buttermilk.
- Avoid skim, nonfat, and low-fat milk.

ATKINS 40 AND ATKINS 100 ACCEPTABLE FOODS

On Atkins 40 and Atkins 100, you can eat all the foods shown previously for Atkins 20, Levels 1 through 4, in addition to the following foods, which are listed with serving sizes that correspond to either 5 grams or 10 grams of Net Carbs (unless otherwise indicated), so that you can easily keep track.

NUTS AND SEEDS AND THEIR BUTTERS

	Serving Size	Grams of Net Carbs*
Almond butter	¼ cup	5.0
Almonds	½ cup	5.0
Brazil nuts	¾ cup	5.0
Cashew butter	1 tablespoon	5.0
Cashews	2 tablespoons	5.0
Coconut, shredded, unsweetened	1 cup	5.0
Hazelnuts	½ cup	5.0
Macadamia nuts	½ cup	5.0
Peanut butter	3 tablespoons	5.0
Peanuts	3 tablespoons	5.0

Pecans	1 cup	5.0
Pine nuts (piñons)	½ cup	5.0
Pistachios	3 tablespoons	5.0
Pumpkin seeds, hulled	½ cup	5.0
Sesame seeds	¼ cup	5.0
Soy "nuts"	3 tablespoons	5.0
Sunflower seeds, hulled	½ cup	5.0
Walnuts, halves	¾ cup	5.0

Rounded

CHEESE AND OTHER DAIRY PRODUCTS AND PLANT MILKS

	Serving Size	Grams of Net Carbs*
Almond milk, plain, unsweetened	1 cup	1.0
Buttermilk	½ cup	5.0*
Cheese, blue	2 tablespoons	0.4
Cheese, Brie	1 ounce	0.1
Cheese, Cheddar	1 ounce	0.4
Cheese, Colby	1 ounce	0.7
Cheese, cottage	½ cup	5.0*
Cheese, cream, full fat, plain	5 tablespoons	5.0*
Cheese, feta	1 ounce	1.2
Cheese, goat (chevre)	1 ounce	0.3
Cheese, Gouda	1 ounce	0.6
Cheese, Havarti	1 ounce	0.0
Cheese, Jarlsberg	1 ounce	1.2
Cheese, Laughing Cow	1 wedge	1.0

Cheese, Mozzarella, whole milk	1 ounce	0.6
Cheese, Parmesan, chunk	1 ounce	0.9
Cheese, Parmesan, grated	1 tablespoon	0.2
Cheese, Romano, chunk	1 ounce	1.0
Cheese, string, whole	1 ounce	1.0
Cheese, Swiss	1 ounce	1.5
Coconut milk, plain, unsweetened	1 cup	1.0
Cream, heavy	¾ cup	5.0*
Cream, sour	¾ cup	5.0*
Milk, whole	½ cup	5.0*
Ricotta, whole milk	¼ cup	2.0
Soy milk, unsweetened, plain	1 cup	2.0
Yogurt, Greek, whole milk, plain, unsweetened	½ cup	5.0

Rounded

LEGUMES

The serving sizes for dried and fresh legumes are the same, but the serving size for dried legumes are for after they are cooked, and the serving size for fresh legumes are for shelled beans.

	Serving Size	Grams of Net Carbs*
Beans, black or turtle	3 tablespoons/½ cup	5.0/10.0
Beans, cannellini	3 tablespoons/½ cup	5.0/10.0
Beans, Great Northern	2 tablespoons/¼ cup	5.0/10.0
Beans, kidney	3 tablespoons/½ cup	5.0/10.0
Beans, Lima	3 tablespoons/½ cup	5.0/10.0
Beans, pinto	3 tablespoons/½ cup	5.0/10.0
Chickpeas/garbanzo beans	2 tablespoons/¼ cup	5.0/10.0

Hummus (plain)	5 tablespoons/⅔ cup	5.0/10.0
Peas, black-eyed	3 tablespoons/½ cup	5.0/10.0
Peas, split	3 tablespoons/½ cup	5.0/10.0
Soybeans, green edamame	10 tablespoons/½ cup	5.0/10.0
Soybeans, white	5 tablespoons/⅔ cup	5.0/10.0

*Rounded

FRUIT

The following carb counts are for fresh fruit.

	Serving Size	Grams of Net Carbs*
Apple	⅓ medium/⅔ medium	5.0/10.0
Apricot	½ medium/1 medium	5.0/10.0
Banana	¼ small/½ small	5.0/10.0
Blackberries	¾ cup/1½ cups	5.0/10.0
Blueberries	¼ cup/½ cup	5.0/10.0
Boysenberries	¾ cup/1½ cups	5.0/10.0
Cherries	3 tablespoons/ 6 tablespoons	5.0/10.0
Clementine, sections	⅔ cup/1⅓ cups	5.0/10.0
Coconut, flaked	1 cup/2 cups	5.0/10.0
Cranberries	⅔ cup/1⅓ cups	5.0/10.0
Dates	1 fruit/2 fruits	5.0/10.0
Fig	¾ small/1½ small	5.0/10.0
Gooseberries	⅓ cup/⅔ cup	5.0/10.0
Grapefruit	¼ medium/½ medium	5.0/10.0
Grapes	3 tablespoons/ 6 tablespoons	5.0/10.0
Guava, sliced	⅓ cup/⅔ cup	5.0/10.0

Kiwi	⅔ medium/1⅓ medium	5.0/10.0
Lemon juice	5 tablespoons/ 10 tablespoons	5.0/10.0
Lime juice	4½ tablespoons/ 9 tablespoons	5.0/10.0
Mango, sliced	¼ cup/½ cup	5.0/10.0
Melon, cantaloupe, balls	½ cup/1 cup	5.0/10.0
Melon, honeydew, balls	⅓ cup/⅔ cup	5.0/10.0
Orange	½ medium/1 medium	5.0/10.0
Peach	½ small/1 small	5.0/10.0
Pear	¼ fruit/½ fruit	5.0/10.0
Pineapple, chunks	¼ cup/½ cup	5.0/10.0
Plum	¾ small/1½ small	5.0/10.0
Raisins	¾ tablespoon/ 1½ tablespoons	5.0/10.0
Raspberries	¾ cup/1½ cups	5.0/10.0
Rhubarb	1½ cups/3 cups	5.0/10.0
Strawberries	½ cup/1 cup	5.0/10.0
Watermelon, balls	½ cup/1 cup	5.0/10.0

Rounded

STARCHY VEGETABLES

All vegetables are measured after cooking.

	Serving Size	Grams of Net Carbs*
Beets	¼ cup/½ cup	5.0/10.0
Carrots, sliced	½ cup/1 cup	5.0/10.0
Corn	¼ cup/½ cup	5.0/10.0
Parsnips	¼ cup/½ cup	5.0/10.0

Peas	¼ cup/½ cup	5.0/10.0
Potato, small, baked	¼ potato/½ potato	5.0/10.0
Rutabaga	½ cup/1 cup	5.0/10.0
Squash, acorn	¼ cup/½ cup	5.0/10.0
Squash, butternut, baked	⅓ cup/⅔ cup	5.0/10.0
Sweet potato, medium, baked	¼ potato/½ potato	5.0/10.0

Rounded

WHOLE GRAINS

	Serving Size	Grams of Net Carbs*
Barley, cooked	2 tablespoons/¼ cup	5.0/10.0
Bread, whole wheat	½ slice/1 slice	5.0/10.0
Coconut flour	2½ tablespoons/⅓ cup	5.0/10.0
Couscous, cooked	2½ tablespoons/⅓ cup	5.0/10.0
Grits, cooked	2½ tablespoons/⅓ cup	5.0/10.0
Millet, cooked	2 tablespoons/¼ cup	5.0/10.0
Oat bran	2 tablespoons/ 4 tablespoons	5.0/10.0
Oatmeal, steel cut	2 tablespoons/¼ cup	5.0/10.0
Pasta, cooked	2½ tablespoons/⅓ cup	5.0/10.0
Polenta	1 tablespoon/ 2 tablespoons	5.0/10.0
Quinoa, cooked	2½ tablespoons/⅓ cup	5.0/10.0
Rice, brown, cooked	2 tablespoons/¼ cup	5.0/10.0
Wheat bran	6 tablespoons/¾ cup	5.0/10.0
Wheat germ	2 tablespoons/¼ cup	5.0/10.0

Rounded

ALCOHOLIC BEVERAGES

	Serving Size	Grams of Net Carbs*
Beer, light	12 ounces	5.6
Beer, low carb	12 ounces	2.5
Bourbon	1 ounce	0.0
Champagne	1 ounce	2.0–3.0
Rum	1 ounce	0.0
Scotch	1 ounce	0.0
Vodka	1 ounce	0.0
Wine, red	3.5 ounces	2.6
Wine, white	3.5 ounces	2.0

Rounded

CLIMBING THE
CARB LADDER

As you move beyond Atkins 20, Level 1, the Carb Ladder will help you in two ways. First, it provides a logical progression with which to add carbohydrate foods once you move beyond the basic foods you can consume on Level 1. Secondly, it prioritizes their amount and frequency. On the lower rungs, you'll see the foods you should be eating most often. On the top rungs are the foods that—even in Level 4—will put in an appearance only occasionally, rarely, or never, depending upon your tolerance for carbs.

People who are relatively tolerant of carbs may be able to introduce some foods in Level 2 that are usually not introduced until Level 3. Other people who are relatively intolerant of carbs may not be able to introduce certain foods coded for Level 2 until Level 3 or Level 4. Again, depending upon their individual tolerance for carbs, some people are able to introduce foods coded for Level 3 and beyond infrequently, in very small quantities, or not at all.

LEVEL 1

Rung 1: Foundation Vegetables: leafy greens and other low-carb vegetables

Rung 2: Dairy foods high in fat and low in carbs: cream, sour cream, and most hard cheeses

LEVEL 2

Rung 3: Nuts and seeds (but not chestnuts)

Rung 4: Berries, cherries, and melon (but not watermelon)

Rung 5: Whole-milk yogurt and fresh cheeses, such as cottage cheese and ricotta

Rung 6: Legumes, including chickpeas, lentils, and the like

Rung 7: Tomato and vegetable juice "cocktail" (plus more lemon and lime juice)

LEVELS 3 AND 4

Rung 8: Other fruits (but not fruit juices or dried fruits)

Rung 9: Higher-carb vegetables, such as winter squash, carrots, and peas

Rung 10: Whole grains

HOW TO REINTRODUCE CERTAIN FOODS

There are five important things to do as you begin to reintroduce foods in Level 2:

1. **Count your Net Carbs.** If you've been estimating grams of Net Carbs while in Level 1, now is the time to start counting them.
2. **Add one food at a time.** Add only one new food within a rung each day or every several days. That way, if a food reawakens cravings or uncontrollable hunger, causes gastric distress, or stalls or reverses your weight loss, you can easily identify it—and back off for the time being. So, for example, at rung 4 you might start with a small portion of blueberries. Assuming you have no problems with that, you can move on to strawberries a couple of days later.

In Level 2, most people can also consume additional low-carb specialty foods beyond those suitable for Level 1. Again, try them one at a time to assess any reactions.

3. **Add more variety, not more food.** You're increasing your range of foods but not the amount of food that you're eating day to day by very much. As you continue to add small amounts of carbohydrate foods, you don't have to do anything other than make sure you're not overdoing your protein intake (typically 4 to 6 ounces at each meal). Let your appetite be your guide. Stay hydrated, and the moment you feel you've had enough, stop eating.

4. **Stay with Foundation Vegetables.** As you add new foods, you'll substitute some of them for other carb foods you're already eating, but not your 12 to 15 grams of Net Carbs from Foundation Vegetables. For example, you can now have cottage cheese in lieu of some of the hard cheese you've been eating in Level 1. Instead of an afternoon snack of green olives, you might switch off with macadamias. You'll still be eating those Level 1–friendly foods, but you can branch out a bit. As long as you're tracking your carb intake, eating the recommended amount of vegetables, and feeling full but not stuffed, you should do fine.

5. **Keep a food journal.** The process of adding back foods doesn't always happen smoothly, and you'll want to know which food is causing which response so, if necessary, you know which to back off from. Keep on noting what you're adding, how much, and your reactions, if any, in your food journal.

SCIENTIFIC REFERENCES

INTRODUCTION

American Diabetes Association. (2018). Economic costs of Diabetes in the U.S. in 2017. *Diabetes Care* 41(5): 917–28.

Centers for Disease Control and Prevention. (2018). Mean macronutrient intake among adults aged 20 and over, by sex and age: United States, selected years 1988–1994 through 2013–2016. Health, United States. Table 56. https://www.cdc.gov/nchs/data/hus/2017/056.pdf.

Cohen, E., Cragg, M., deFonseka, J., Hite, A., Rosenberg, M., and Zhou, B. (2015). Statistical review of US macronutrient consumption data, 1965–2011: Americans have been following dietary guidelines, coincident with the rise in obesity. *Nutrition* 31(5): 727–32.

Dong, T., Guo, M., Zhang, P., Sun, G., and Chen, B. (2020). The effects of low-carbohydrate diets on cardiovascular risk factors: a meta-analysis. *PLOS ONE* 15(1): e0225348.

Evert, A. B., Dennison, M., Gardner, C. D., Garvey, W. T., Lau, K. H. K., MacLeod, J., et al. (2019). Nutrition therapy for adults with diabetes or prediabetes: a consensus report. *Diabetes Care* 42(5): 731–54.

Fryar, C. D., Carroll, M .D., and Ogden, C. L. (2018). Prevalence of overweight, obesity, and severe obesity among adults aged 20 and over: United States, 1960–1962 through 2015–2016. *Health E-Stats*, National Center for Health Statistics, Centers for Disease Control and Prevention.

Gross, L. S., Li, L., Ford, E. S., and Liu, S. (2004). Increased consumption of refined carbohydrates and the epidemic of type 2 diabetes in the United States: an ecologic assessment. *American Journal of Clinical Nutrition* 79(5): 774–79.

Hallberg, S. J., McKenzie, A. L., Williams, P. T., Bhanpuri, N. H., Peters, A. L., et al. (2018). Effectiveness and safety of a novel care model for the management of type 2 diabetes at 1 year: an open-label, non-randomized, controlled study. *Diabetes Therapy* 9(2): 583–612.

Menke, A., Casagrande, S., Geiss, L., and Cowie, C. C. (2015). Prevalence of and trends in diabetes among adults in the United States, 1988–2012. *Journal of the American Medical Association* 314(10): 1021–29.

Saslow, L. R., Daubenmier, J. J., Moskowitz, J. T., Kim, S., Murphy, E. J., Phinney, S.D., et al. (2017). Twelve-month outcomes of a randomized trial of a moderate-carbohydrate versus very low-carbohydrate diet in overweight adults with type 2 diabetes mellitus or prediabetes. *Nutrition & Diabetes* 7(12): 304.

United States Department of Agriculture. (2015). Dietary guidelines for Americans, 2015–2020. https://health.gov/sites/default/files/2019-09/2015-2020_Dietary_Guidelines.pdf.

Ward, Z. J., Bleich, S. N., Cradock, A. L., Barrett, J. L., Giles, G. M., Flax, C., et al. (2019). Projected U.S. state-level prevalence of adult obesity and severe obesity. *The New England Journal of Medicine* 381(25): 2440–50.

CHAPTER 1

Abdelhamid, A. S., Brown, T. S., Brainard, J. S., Biswas, P., Thorpe, G. C., Moore, H. J., et al. (2020). Omega-3 fatty acids for the primary and secondary prevention of cardiovascular disease. *Cochrane Database of Systematic Reviews* 3: CD003177.

Aguilar, M., Bhuket, T., Torres, S., Liu, B., and Wong, R. J. (2015). Prevalence of the metabolic syndrome in the United States, 2003–2012. *Journal of the American Medical Association* 313(19): 1973–74.

Arpaia, N., Campell, C., Fan, X., Dikiy, S., van der Veeken, J., deRoos, P., et al. (2013). Metabolites produced by commensal bacteria promote peripheral regulatory T-cell generation. *Nature* 504(7480): 451–55.

Bush, N. C., Resuehr, H. E. S., Goree, L. L., Locher, J. L., Bray, M. S., Soleymani, T., et al. (2018). A high-fat compared with a high-carbohydrate breakfast enhances 24-hour fat oxidation in older adults. *Journal of Nutrition* 148(2): 220–26.

Calder, P. C. (2017). Omega-3 fatty acids and inflammatory processes: from molecules to man. *Biochemical Society Transactions* 45(5): 1105–15.

Chen, S. C., Lin, Y. H., Huang, H. P., Hsu, W. L., Houng, J. Y., Huang, C. K. (2012). Effect of conjugated linoleic acid supplementation on weight loss and body fat composition in a Chinese population. *Nutrition* 28(5): 559–65.

Cohen, C. W., Fontaine, K. R., Arend, R.C., Soleymani, T., and Gower, B. A. (2018). Favorable effects of a ketogenic diet on physical function, perceived energy, and food cravings in women with ovarian or endometrial cancer: a randomized, controlled trial. *Nutrients* 10(9): 1187.

Cummings, J. H., Pomare, E. W., Branch, W. J., Naylor, C. P., and Macfarlane, G. T. (1987). Short chain fatty acids in human large intestine, portal, hepatic and venous blood. *Gut* 28(10): 1221–27.

Dashti, H. M., Mathew, T. C., Khadada, M., Al-Mousawi, M., Talib, H., Asfar, S. K., et al. (2007). Beneficial effects of ketogenic diet in obese diabetic subjects. *Molecular and Cellular Biochemistry* 302(1–2): 249–56.

Emery, S., Haberling, I., Berger, G., Walitza, S., Schmeck, K., Albert, T., et al. (2020). Omega-3 and its domain-specific effects on cognitive test performance in youths: a meta-analysis. *Neuroscience & Biobehavioral Reviews* 112: 420–36.

Gaullier, J. M., Halse, J., Hoivik, H. O., Hoye, K., Syvertsen, C., Nurminiemi M., et al. (2007). Six months supplementation with conjugated linoleic acid induces regional-specific fat mass decreases in overweight and obese. *British Journal of Nutrition* 97(3): 550–60.

Gibson, G. R., and Roberfroid, M. B. (1995). Dietary modulation of the human colonic microbiota: introducing the concept of prebiotics. *Journal of Nutrition* 125(6): 1401–12.

Hyde, P. N., Sapper, T. N., Crabtree, C. D., LaFountain, R. A., Bowling, M. L., Buga, A., et al. (2019). Dietary carbohydrate restriction improves metabolic syndrome independent of weight loss. *JCI Insight* 4(12): e128308.

Iacovides, S., Goble, D., Paterson, B., and Meiring, R. M. (2019). Three consecutive weeks of nutritional ketosis has no effect on cognitive function, sleep, and mood compared with a high-carbohydrate, low-fat diet in healthy individuals: a randomized, crossover, controlled trial. *American Journal of Clinical Nutrition* 110(2): 349–57.

Johnstone, A. M. Horgan, G. W., Murison, S. D., Bremner, D. M., and Lobley, G. E. (2008). Effects of a high-protein ketogenic diet on hunger, appetite, and weight loss in obese men feeding ad libitum. *American Journal of Clinical Nutrition* 87(1): 44–55.

Kossoff, E. H., Zupec-Kania, B. A., Auvin, S., Ballaban-Gil, K. R., Christina Bergqvist, A. G., Blackford, R., et al. (2018). Optimal clinical management of children receiving dietary therapies for epilepsy: updated recommendations of the International Ketogenic Diet Study Group. *Epilepsia Open* 3(2): 175–92.

Liao, Y., Xie, B., Zhang, H., He, Q., Guo, L., Subramaniapillai, M., et al. (2019). Efficacy of omega-3 PUFAs in depression: a meta-analysis. *Translational Psychiatry* 9(1): 190.

Martin, C. K., Rosenbaum, D., Han, H., Geiselman, P. J., Wyatt, H. R., Hill, J. O., et al. (2011). Change in food cravings, food preferences, and appetite during a low-carbohydrate and low-fat diet. *Obesity* 19(10): 1963–70.

McClernon, F. J., Yancy, W. S. Jr., Eberstein, J. A., Atkins, R. C., Westman, E. C. (2007). The effects of a low-carbohydrate ketogenic diet and a low-fat diet on mood, hunger, and other self-reported symptoms. *Obesity* 15(1): 182–87.

Piers, L. S., Walker, K. Z., Stoney, R. M., Soares, M. J., and O'Dea, K. (2002). The influence of the type of dietary fat on postprandial fat oxidation rates: monounsaturated (olive oil) *vs* saturated fat (cream). *International Journal of Obesity and Related Metabolic Disorders* 26(6): 814–21.

Samaha, F. F., Iqbal, N., Seshadri, P., Chicano, K. L., Daily, D. A., McGrory, J., et al. (2003). A low-carbohydrate as compared with a low-fat diet in severe obesity. *New England Journal of Medicine* 348(21): 2074–81.

Sharman, M. J., Gomez, A. L., Kraemer, W. J., Volek, J. S. (2004). Very low-carbohydrate and low-fat diets affect fasting lipids and postprandial lipemia differently in overweight men. *Journal of Nutrition* 134(4): 880–85.

Siegmann, M. J., Athinarayanan, S. J., Hallberg, S. J., McKenzie, A. L., Bhanpuri, N. H., Campell, W. W., et al. (2019). Improvement in patient-reported sleep in type 2 diabetes and prediabetes participants receiving a continuous care intervention with nutritional ketosis. *Sleep Medicine* 55: 92–99.

Slavin, J. (2013). Fiber and prebiotics: mechanisms and health benefits. *Nutrients* 5(4): 1417–35.

Stavrinou, P. S., Andreou, E., Aphamis, G., Pantzaris, M., Ioannou, M., Patrikios, I.S., et al. (2020). The effects of a 6-month high dose omega-3 and omega-6 polyunsaturated fatty acids and antioxidant vitamins supplementation on cognitive function and functional capacity in older adults with mild cognitive impairment. *Nutrients* 12(2): 325.

Syvertsen, C., Halse, J., Hoivik, H. O., Gaulier, J. M., Nurminiemi, M., Kristiansen, K., et al. (2007). The effect of 6 months supplementation with conjugated linoleic acid on insulin resistance in overweight and obese. *International Journal of Obesity* 31(7): 1148–54.

Trompette, A., Gollwitzer, W. S., Yadava, K., Sichelstiel, A. K., Sprenger, N., Ngom-Bru, C., et al. (2014). Gut microbiota metabolism of dietary fiber influences allergic airway disease and hematopoiesis. *Nature Medicine* 20(2): 159–66.

Vanegas, S. M., Meydani, M., Barnett, J. B., Goldin, B., Kane, A., Rasmussen, H., et al. (2017). Substituting whole grains for refined grains in a 6-wk randomized trial has a modest effect on gut microbiota and immune and inflammatory markers of healthy adults. *American Journal of Clinical Nutrition* 105(3): 635–50.

Volek, J. S., Freidenreich, D. J., Saenz, C., Kunces, L. J., Creighton, B. C., Bartley, J. M., et al. (2016). Metabolic characteristics of keto-adapted ultra-endurance runners. *Metabolism* 65(3): 100–10.

Volek, J. S., Sharman, M., Gomez, A., Judelson, D., Rubin, M., Watson, G., et al. (2004). Comparison of energy-restricted very low-carbohydrate and low-fat diets on weight loss and body composition in overweight men and women. *Nutrition & Metabolism* 1(1): 13.

Zhou, W., Mukherjee, P., Kiebish, M. A., Markis, W. T., Mantis, J. G., and Seyfried, T. N. (2007). The calorically restricted ketogenic diet, an effective alternative therapy for malignant brain cancer. *Nutrition & Metabolism* 4: 5.

CHAPTER 2

Anguah, K. O., Syed-Abdul, M. M., Hu, Q., Jacome-Sosa, M., Heimowitz, C., Cox, V., et al. (2019). Changes in food cravings and eating behavior after a dietary carbohydrate restriction intervention trial. *Nutrients* 12(1): 52.

Aune, D., Giovannucci, E., Boffetta, P., Fadnes, L. T., Keum, N., Norat, T., et al. (2017). Fruit and vegetable intake and the risk of cardiovascular disease, total cancer and all-cause mortality—a systematic review and dose-response meta-analysis of prospective studies. *International Journal of Epidemiology* 46(3): 1029–56.

Ebbeling, C. B., Feldman, H. A., Klein, G. L., Wong, J. M. W., Bielak, L., Steltz, S. K., et al. (2018). Effects of a low carbohydrate diet on energy expenditure during weight loss maintenance: randomized trial. *BMJ* 363: k4583.

Fothergill, E., Guo, J., Howard, L., Kerns, J. C., Knuth, N. D., Brychta, R., et al. (2016). Persistent metabolic adaptation 6 years after "The Biggest Loser" competition. *Obesity* 24(8): 1612–19.

Heffron, S. P., Rockman, C. B., Adelman, M. A., Gianos, E., Guo, Y., Xu, J. F., et al. (2017). Greater frequency of fruit and vegetable consumption is associated with lower prevalence of peripheral artery disease. *Arteriosclerosis, Thrombosis, and Vascular Biology* 37(6): 1234–40.

Hollis, J. F., Gullion, C. M., Stevens, V. J., Brantley, P. J., Appel, L. J., Ard, J. D., et al. (2008). Weight loss during the intensive intervention phase of the weight-loss maintenance trial. *American Journal of Preventive Medicine* 35(2): 118–26.

Lapuente, M., Estruch, R., Shahbaz, M., and Casas, R. (2019). Relation of fruits and vegetables with major cardiometabolic risk factors, markers of oxidation, and inflammation. *Nutrients* 11(10): 2381.

Martin, C. K., Rosenbaum, D., Han, H., Geiselman, P. J., Wyatt, H. R., Hill, J. O., et al. (2011). Change in food cravings, food preferences, and appetite during a low-carbohydrate and low-fat diet. *Obesity* 19(10): 1963–70.

McClernon, F. J., Yancy, W. S. Jr., Eberstein, J. A., Atkins, R. C., and Westman, E. C. (2007). The effects of a low-carbohydrate ketogenic diet and a low-fat diet on mood, hunger, and other self-reported symptoms. *Obesity* 15(1): 182–87.

Navarro, S. L., Schwarz, Y., Song, X., Wang, C. Y., Chen, C., Trudo, S. P., et al. (2014). Cruciferous vegetables have variable effects on biomarkers of systemic inflammation in a randomized controlled trial in healthy young adults. *Journal of Nutrition* 144(11): 1850–57.

CHAPTER 3

American Heart Association. (2018). American Heart Association recommendations for physical activity in adults and kids. https://www.heart.org/en/healthy-living/fitness/fitness-basics/aha-recs-for-physical-activity-in-adults.

Aune, D., Norat, T., Leitzmann, M., Tonstad, S., and Vatten, L. J. (2015). Physical activity and the risk of type 2 diabetes: a systematic review and dose-response meta-analysis. *European Journal of Epidemiology* 30(7): 529–42.

Blackwell, D. L., and Clarke, T. C. (2018). State variation in meeting the 2008 federal guidelines for both aerobic and muscle-strengthening activities through leisure-time physical activity among adults aged 18–64: United States, 2010–2015. *National Health Statistics Reports* 112: 1–22.

Chiu, S., Bergeron, N., Williams, P. T., Bray, G. A., Sutherland, B., and Krauss, R. M. (2016). Comparison of the DASH (Dietary Approaches to Stop Hypertension) diet and a higher-fat DASH diet on blood pressure and lipids and lipoproteins: a randomized controlled trial. *American Journal of Clinical Nutrition* 103(2): 341–47.

Dugan, S. A., Bromberger, J. T., Segawa, E., Avery, E., and Sternfeld, B. (2015). Association between physical activity and depressive symptoms: midlife women in SWAN. *Medicine & Science in Sports & Exercise* 47(2): 335–42.

Ekelund, U., Brown, W. J., Steene-Johannessen, J., Fagerland, M. W., Owen, N., Powell, K. E., et al. (2019). Do the associations of sedentary behaviour with cardiovascular disease mortality and cancer mortality differ by physical activity level? A systematic review and harmonised meta-analysis of data from 850,060 participants. *British Journal of Sports Medicine* 53(14): 886–94.

Ekelund, U., Tarp, J., Steene-Johannessen, J., Hansen, B. H., Jefferis, B., Fagerland, M. W., et al., (2019). Dose-response associations between accelerometry measured physical activity and sedentary time and all cause mortality: systematic review and harmonised meta-analysis. *BMJ* 366: l4570.

Gomes, W. R., Devoz, P. P., Araujo, M. L., Batista, B. L., Barbosa, F. Jr., and Barcelos, G. R., M. et al. (2017). Milk and dairy products intake is associated with low levels of lead (Pb) in workers highly exposed to the metal. *Biological Trace Element Research* 178(1): 29–35.

Kephart, W. C., Pledge, C. D., Roberson, P. A., Mumford, P. W., Romero, M. A., Mobley, C. B., et al. (2018). The three-month effects of a ketogenic diet on body composition, blood parameters, and performance metrics in CrossFit trainees: a pilot study. *Sports* 6(1): 1.

Knab, A. M., Shanely, R. A., Corbin, K. D., Jin, F., Sha, W., and Nieman, D. C. (2011). A 45-minute vigorous exercise bout increases metabolic rate for 14 hours. *Medicine & Science in Sports & Exercise* 43(9): 1643–48.

Lachman, S., Boekholdt, S. M., Luben, R. N., Sharp, S. J., Brage, S., Khaw, K. T., et al. (2018). Impact of physical activity on the risk of cardiovascular disease in middle-aged and older adults: EPIC Norfolk prospective population study. *European Journal of Preventive Cardiology* 25(2): 200–08.

LaFountain, R. A., Miller, V. J., Barnhart, E. C., Hyde, P. N., Crabtree, C. D., McSwiney, F. T., et al. (2019). Extended ketogenic diet and physical training intervention in military personnel. *Military Medicine* 184(9–10): e538–47.

Rodriguez-Gomez, I., Manas, A., Losa-Reyna, J., Rodriguez-Manas, L., Chastin, F. F. M., Alegre, L. M., et al. (2018). Associations between sedentary time, physical activity and bone health among older people using compositional data analysis. *PLOS ONE* 13(10): e0206013.

Schoenfeld, B. J., and Aragon, A. A. (2018). How much protein can the body use in a single meal for muscle-building? Implications for daily protein distribution. *Journal of the International Society of Sports Nutrition* 15: 10.

Schoenfeld, B. J., Aragon, A., Wilborn, C., Urbina, S. L., Hayward, S. E., and Krieger, J. (2017). Pre- versus post-exercise protein intake has similar effects on muscular adaptations. *PeerJ* 5: e2825.

Schwalfenberg, G. K., and Genuis, S. J. (2015). Vitamin D, essential minerals, and toxic elements: exploring interactions between nutrients and toxicants in clinical medicine. *Scientific World Journal* 2015: article 318595.

Strasser, B. (2013). Physical activity in obesity and metabolic syndrome. *Annals of the New York Academy of Sciences* 1281: 141–59.

van der Berg, J. D., Stehouwer, C. D., Bosma, H., van der Velde, J. H., Willems, P. J., Savelberg, H. H., et al. (2016). Associations of total amount and patterns of sedentary behaviour with type 2 diabetes and the metabolic syndrome: the Maastricht Study. *Diabetologia* 59(4): 709–18.

Volek, J. S., Freidenreich, D. J., Saenz, C., Kunces, L. J., Creighton, B. C., Bartley, J. M., et al. (2016). Metabolic characteristics of keto-adapted ultra-endurance runners. *Metabolism* 65(3): 100–10.

Waldman, H. S., Smith, J. W., Lamberth, J., Fountain, B. J., and McAllister, M. J. (2019). A 28-day carbohydrate-restricted diet improves markers of cardiometabolic health and performance in professional firefighters. *Journal of Strength & Conditioning Research* 33(12): 3284–94.

Wood, R. J., and M. L. Fernandez. (2009). Carbohydrate-restricted versus low-glycemic-index diets for the treatment of insulin resistance and metabolic syndrome. *Nutrition Reviews* 67(3): 179–83.

CHAPTER 4

Birt, D. F., Boylson, T., Hendrich, S., Jane, J. L., Hollis, J., Li, L. et al. (2013). Resistant starch: promise for improving human health. *Advances in Nutrition* 4(6): 587–601.

Chiu, Y. T., and Stewart, M. L. (2013). Effect of variety and cooking method on resistant starch content of white rice and subsequent postprandial glucose response and appetite in humans. *Asia Pacific Journal of Clinical Nutrition* 22(3): 372–79.

Hung, P. V., Vien, N. L., and Lan Phi, N. T. (2016). Resistant starch improvement of rice starches under a combination of acid and heat-moisture treatments. *Food Chemistry* 191: 67–73.

Rickman, J. C., Barrett, D. M., and Bruhn, C. M. (2007). Nutritional comparison of fresh, frozen and canned fruits and vegetables. Part 1. Vitamins C and B and phenolic compounds. *Journal of the Science of Food and Agriculture* 87(6): 930–44.

CHAPTER 5

Blesso, C. N., Andersen, C. J., Barona, J., Volk, B., Volek, J. S., Fernandez, M. L. (2013). Effects of carbohydrate restriction and dietary cholesterol provided by eggs on clinical risk factors in metabolic syndrome. *Journal of Clinical Lipidology* 7(5): 463–71.

Fernandez, M. L. (2006). Dietary cholesterol provided by eggs and plasma lipoproteins in healthy populations. *Current Opinion in Clinical Nutrition & Metabolic Care* 9(1): 8–12.

Forsythe, C. E., Phinney, S. D., Feinman, R. D., Volk, B. M., Freidenreich, D., Quann, E., et al. (2010). Limited effect of dietary saturated fat on plasma saturated fat in the context of a low carbohydrate diet. *Lipids* 45(10): 947–62.

Zeraatkar, D., Johnston, B. C., Bartoszko, J., Cheung, K., Bala, M. M., valli, C., et al. (2019). Effect of lower versus higher red meat intake on cardiometabolic and cancer outcomes: a systematic review of randomized trials. *Annals of Internal Medicine* 171(10): 721–31.

CHAPTER 6

Hajishafiee, M., Bitarafan, V., and Feinle-Bisset, C. (2019). Gastrointestinal sensing of meal-related signals in humans, and dysregulations in eating-related disorders. *Nutrients* 11(6): 1298.

Parretti, H. M., Aveyard, P., Balnnin, A., Clifford, S. J., Coleman, S. J., Roalfe, A., et al. (2015). Efficacy of water preloading before main meals as a strategy for weight loss in primary care patients with obesity: RCT. *Obesity* 23(9): 1785–91.

Reed, M. O., Aiy, Y., Leutcher, J. L., and Jane, J. L. (2013). Effects of cooking methods and starch structures on starch hydrolysis rates of rice. *Journal of Food Science* 78(7): H1076–81.

Truth about dining out. (2019). Fourth. https://www.fourth.com/wp-content/uploads/2019/10/US_Infographic_Truth-About-Dining-Out_102919.pdf.

CHAPTER 7

Auestad, N., and Fulgoni, V. L., III. (2015). What current literature tells us about sustainable diets: emerging research linking dietary patterns, environmental sustainability, and economics. *Advances in Nutrition* 6(1): 19–36.

Christen, W. G., Liu, S., Glynn, R. J., Gaziano, J. M., and Buring, J. E. (2008). Dietary carotenoids, vitamins C and E, and risk of cataract in women: a prospective study. *Archives of Ophthalmology* 126(1): 102–9.

Gerber, P. J., Steinfeld, H., Henderson, B., Mottet, A., Opio, C., Dijkman, J., et al. (2013). Tackling climate change through livestock: A global assessment of emissions and mitigation opportunities. Food and Agriculture Organization of the United Nations. http://www.fao.org/3/a-i3437e.pdf.

Jia, Y. P., Sun, L., Yu, H. S., Liang, L. P., Li, W., Ding, H., et al. (2017). The pharmacological effects of lutein and zeaxanthin on visual disorders and cognition diseases. *Molecules* 22(4): 610.

Jiang, X., Huang, J., Song, D., Deng, R., Wei, J., and Zhang, Z. (2017). Increased consumption of fruit and vegetables is related to a reduced risk of cognitive impairment and dementia: meta-analysis. *Frontiers in Aging Neuroscience* 9: 18.

Moeller, S. M., Voland, R., Tinker, L., Blodi, B. A., Klein, M. L., et al. (2008). Associations between age-related nuclear cataract and lutein and zeaxanthin in the diet and serum in the Carotenoids in the Age-Related Eye Disease Study, an ancillary study of the Women's Health Initiative. *Archives of Ophthalmology* 126(3): 354–64.

Murray, I. J., Makridaki, M., van der Veen, R. L., Carden, D., Parry, N. R., and Berendschot, T. T. (2013). Lutein supplementation over a one-year period in early AMD might have a mild beneficial effect on visual acuity: the CLEAR study. *Investigative Ophthalmology & Visual Science* 54(3): 1781–78.

Richer, S., Stiles, W., Statkute, L., Pulido, J., Frankowski, J., Rudy, D., et al., (2004). Double-masked, placebo-controlled, randomized trial of lutein and antioxidant supplementation in the intervention of atrophic age-related macular degeneration: the Veterans LAST study (Lutein Antioxidant Supplementation Trial). *Optometry* 75(4): 216–30.

Wang, Y., Li, F., Wang, Z., Qiu, T., Shen, Y., and Wang, M. (2015). Fruit and vegetable consumption and risk of lung cancer: a dose-response meta-analysis of prospective cohort studies. *Lung Cancer* 88(2): 124–30.

Wu, Y., Zhang, D., Jiang, X., and Jiang, W. (2015). Fruit and vegetable consumption and risk of type 2 diabetes mellitus: a dose-response meta-analysis of prospective cohort studies. *Nutrition, Metabolism & Cardiovascular Diseases* 25(2): 140–47.

Zhan, J., Liu, Y. J., Cai, L. B., Xu, F. R., Xie, T., and He, Q. Q. (2017). Fruit and vegetable consumption and risk of cardiovascular disease: a meta-analysis of prospective cohort studies. *Critical Reviews in Food Science and Nutrition* 57(8): 1650–63.

ACKNOWLEDGMENTS

YOU CAN ACHIEVE GREAT THINGS with a team that you can't achieve alone. I'm proud to say that writing this book was indeed a team effort. It began with the realization that we had this amazing opportunity to speak to you about embracing a better way of eating by learning how to live Atkins 100's low-carb lifestyle, because you are passionate about the food you eat and how it impacts your overall health and wellness. You aren't interested in a short-term "fix" but an eating solution such as Atkins 100 that you can embrace and sustain, with a personalized approach.

I am thankful to the leadership and vision of Scott Parker, Chief Marketing Officer at Simply Good Foods Company, and Jennifer Livingston, Director of Communications, who were enormously helpful with insightful comments and additions from the very beginning and through the continual process of bringing this book to life. Gretchen Ferraro, our Editorial Director, collaborated with me, and without her contributions, this second book that we've worked on together would not have been possible. Jonathan Clinthorne, Ph.D., our Nutrition Communication Manager, pored over every word for nutritional accuracy and supplied scientific references and insight whenever we needed it. Lani Banner, our nutritionist and recipe developer, created our delicious and useful meal plans, which incorporated the recipes in this book. She also cooked and tested every recipe in the book, which brought smiles to all the "unofficial" taste testers in our Denver office. It was no easy task to meet all our nutritional targets, but she did it. And I would like to extend a special thanks to Joe Scalzo, Chief Executive Officer at Simply Good Foods Company, for his insights in supporting this book and assembling this talented team.

The key to this book are the mouthwatering low-carb and low-sugar recipes created by Mindy Fox. Thanks to Mindy's finely tuned recipe development and creativity, we are able to demonstrate once and for all that eating the Atkins 100 way is wonderfully flexible and can be personalized to suit your individual needs. With Atkins, food should be an experience worth sharing and savoring with others, and these recipes are a testament to that.

Finally, this book would not have been possible without Joy Tutela, from the David Black Literary Agency, who went above and beyond in coordinating the moving pieces, publisher Libby McGuire, who assembled a talented team that was a pleasure to work with, the superb editorial efforts of Leah Miller, executive editor at Atria/Simon & Schuster, and Melanie Iglesias Perez for her careful shepherding of the book throughout the entire process.